William C. Gaventa, Jr., MDiv
David L. Coulter, MD
Editors

Spirituality and Intellectual Disability: International Perspectives on the Effect of Culture and Religion on Healing Body, Mind, and Soul

Spirituality and Intellectual Disability: International Perspectives on the Effect of Culture and Religion on Healing Body, Mind, and Soul has been co-published simultaneously as *Journal of Religion, Disability & Health*, Volume 5, Numbers 2/3 2001.

Pre-publication
REVIEWS,
COMMENTARIES,
EVALUATIONS . . .

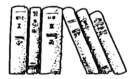

"**M**UST READING for all who believe that people with mental retardation, no matter where they live, have a right to a full life of faith. . . . A VARIETY OF PERSPECTIVES, FROM MANY FAITHS AND CULTURES, on the unique spiritual needs and gifts of people with mental retardation."

Ginny Thornburgh, EdM
Director
Religion and Disability Program
National Organization on Disability
Washington, DC

"Written by Christians, Jews, Muslims, and Native Americans from a variety of locales around the world, the approaches are varied but the message of inclusion is universal. With articles ranging from philosophical considerations to practical strategies to provide access to the rituals and celebrations of Jewish, Christian, Islamic, and other religious practices, this book would be A VALUABLE ASSET IN THE TRAINING OF ALL POTENTIAL 'SPIRITUAL CLINICIANS,' a group that includes not just members of the clergy but also social workers, psychologists, psychiatrists, and physicians."

Becca Hornstein
Executive Director
Council for Jews with Special Needs
Phoenix, AZ

"COMPULSORY READING. . . . Explores the relationship between disability and theology with clarity, commitment, and passion. It is a vital resource for researchers, pastors, and others who seek to understand the everyday practical theology of their calling."

Dr. John Swinton
Department of Divinity
and Religious Studies
King's College
University of Aberdeen
Scotland

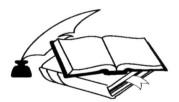

"**A** JOURNEY OF DISCOVERY. . . .
Speaks directly to the abilities
of those who are disabled and to the
deep and abiding relationship which
persons with disabilities have with
the God who created us all."

The Rev. Barbara Ramnaraine
Coordinator
The Episcopal Disability Network
Minneapolis, MN

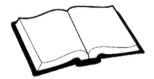

The Haworth Pastoral Press
An Imprint of
The Haworth Press, Inc.
New York • London • Oxford

Spirituality
and Intellectual Disability:
International Perspectives
on the Effect
of Culture and Religion
on Healing Body, Mind, and Soul

Spirituality and Intellectual Disability: International Perspectives on the Effect of Culture and Religion on Healing Body, Mind, and Soul has been co-published simultaneously as *Journal of Religion, Disability & Health*, Volume 5, Numbers 2/3 2001.

The *Journal of Religion, Disability & Health* Monographic "Separates"

(formerly the Journal of Religion in Disability & Rehabilitation series)*

Below is a list of " separates," which in serials librarianship means a special issue simultaneously published as a special journal issue or double-issue *and* as a "separate" hardbound monograph. (This is a format which we also call a "DocuSerial.")

"Separates" are published because specialized libraries or professionals may wish to purchase a specific thematic issue by itself in a format which can be separately cataloged and shelved, as opposed to purchasing the journal on an on-going basis. Faculty members may also more easily consider a "separate" for classroom adoption.

"Separates" are carefully classified separately with the major book jobbers so that the journal tie-in can be noted on new book order slips to avoid duplicate purchasing.

You may wish to visit Haworth's Website at . . .

http://www.HaworthPress.com

. . . to search our online catalog for complete tables of contents of these separates and related publications.

You may also call 1-800-HAWORTH (outside US/Canada: 607-722-5857), or Fax 1-800-895-0582 (outside US/Canada: 607-771-0012), or e-mail at:

getinfo@haworthpressinc.com

Spirituality and Intellectual Disability: International Perspectives on the Effect of Culture and Religion on Healing Body, Mind, and Soul, edited by William C. Gaventa, Jr., MDiv, and David L. Coulter, MD (Vol. 5, No. 2/3, 2001). *"Must reading . . . perspectives from many faiths and cultures on the spiritual needs and gifts of people with mental retardation." (Ginny Thornburgh, EdM, Director, Religion and Disability Program, National Organization on Disability, Washington, DC)*

The Theological Voice of Wolf Wolfensberger, edited by William C. Gaventa, Jr., MDiv, and David L. Coulter, MD (Vol. 4, No. 2/3, 2001). *This thought-provoking volume presents Wolfensberger's challenging, outrageous, and inspiring ideas on the theological significance of disabilities, including the problem with wheelchair access ramps in churches, the meaning of suffering, and the spiritual gifts of the mentally retarded.*

A Look Back: The Birth of the Americans with Disabilities Act, edited by Robert C. Anderson, MDiv (Vol. 2, No. 4, 1996).* *Takes you to the unique moment in American history when persons of many different backgrounds and with different disabilities united to press Congress for full recognition and protection of their rights as American citizens.*

Pastoral Care of the Mentally Disabled: Advancing Care of the Whole Person, edited by Sally K. Severino, MD, and Reverend Richard Liew, PhD (Vol. 1, No. 2, 1994).* *"A great book for theologians with a refreshing dogma-free approach; thought provoking for physiotherapists and all other human beings!" (The Chartered Society of Physiotherapy)*

Spirituality and Intellectual Disability: International Perspectives on the Effect of Culture and Religion on Healing Body, Mind, and Soul

William C. Gaventa, Jr., MDiv
David L. Coulter, MD
Editors

Spirituality and Intellectual Disability: International Perspectives on the Effect of Culture and Religion on Healing Body, Mind, and Soul has been co-published simultaneously as *Journal of Religion, Disability & Health*, Volume 5, Numbers 2/3 2001.

The Haworth Pastoral Press
An Imprint of
The Haworth Press, Inc.
New York • London • Oxford

Published by

The Haworth Pastoral Press, 10 Alice Street, Binghamton, NY 13904-1580 USA

The Haworth Pastoral Press is an imprint of The Haworth Press, Inc., 10 Alice Street, Binghamton, NY 13904-1580 USA.

Spirituality and Intellectual Disability: International Perspectives on the Effect of Culture and Religion on Healing Body, Mind, and Soul has been co-published simultaneously as *Journal of Religion, Disability & Health*, Volume 5, Numbers 2/3 2001.

The development, preparation, and publication of this work has been undertaken with great care. However, the publisher, employees, editors, and agents of The Haworth Press and all imprints of The Haworth Press, Inc., including The Haworth Medical Press® and The Pharmaceutical Products Press®, are not responsible for any errors contained herein or for consequences that may ensue from use of materials or information contained in this work. Opinions expressed by the author(s) are not necessarily those of The Haworth Press, Inc.

Cover design by Thomas J. Mayshock Jr.

Library of Congress Cataloging-in-Publication Data

International Association for the Scientific Study of Intellectual Disabilities. Congress (2000 : Seattle, Wash.)
Spirituality and intellectual disability: international perspectives on the effect of culture and religion on healing body, mind, and soul / William C. Gaventa, Jr., and David L. Coulter, editors.
   p. cm.
  "Co-published simultaneously as Journal of Religion, Disability & Health, volume 5, numbers 2/3 2001."
  Includes bibliographical references and index.
  ISBN 0-7890-1684-2 (hard : alk. paper)–ISBN 0-7890-1685-0 (pbk: alk. paper)
  1. People with mental disabilities–Religious life–Congresses. 2. Mental retardation–Religious aspects–Congresses. I. Gaventa, William C. II. Coulter, David L. III. Title.

BL625.9.P46 I58 2002
291.1′78323–dc21
                          2001059407

Indexing, Abstracting & Website/Internet Coverage

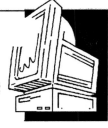

This section provides you with a list of major indexing & abstracting services. That is to say, each service began covering this periodical during the year noted in the right column. Most Websites which are listed below have indicated that they will either post, disseminate, compile, archive, cite or alert their own Website users with research-based content from this work. (This list is as current as the copyright date of this publication.)

(continued)

Special Bibliographic Notes related to special journal issues (separates) and indexing/abstracting:

- indexing/abstracting services in this list will also cover material in any "separate" that is co-published simultaneously with Haworth's special thematic journal issue or DocuSerial. Indexing/abstracting usually covers material at the article/chapter level.
- monographic co-editions are intended for either non-subscribers or libraries which intend to purchase a second copy for their circulating collections.
- monographic co-editions are reported to all jobbers/wholesalers/approval plans. The source journal is listed as the "series" to assist the prevention of duplicate purchasing in the same manner utilized for books-in-series.
- to facilitate user/access services all indexing/abstracting services are encouraged to utilize the co-indexing entry note indicated at the bottom of the first page of each article/chapter/contribution.
- this is intended to assist a library user of any reference tool (whether print, electronic, online, or CD-ROM) to locate the monographic version if the library has purchased this version but not a subscription to the source journal.
- individual articles/chapters in any Haworth publication are also available through the Haworth Document Delivery Service (HDDS).

Spirituality and Intellectual Disability: International Perspectives on the Effect of Culture and Religion on Healing Body, Mind, and Soul

CONTENTS

ABOUT THE EDITORS

William C. Gaventa, Jr., MDiv, is Coordinator of Community and Congregational Supports at the Elizabeth M. Boggs Center of Developmental Disabilities, the University Affiliated Program of New Jersey. He also coordinates a training and technical assistance team for the New Jersey Self Determination Initiative, which now supports more than 125 individuals and their families. Mr. Gaventa also served as Coordinator of Family Support for the Georgia Developmental Disabilities Council, Chaplain and Coordinator of Religious Services for the Monroe Developmental Center, and Executive Secretary for the Religion Division of the AAMR since 1985. He completed a term on the Board of Directors of the AAMR, and serves on the Board of the National Federation of Interfaith Volunteer Caregivers. He is co-editor of *The Theological Voice of Wolf Wolfensberger* (Haworth).

David L. Coulter, MD, is a member of the faculty of the Departments of Neurology and Social Medicine at Harvard Medical School and is affiliated with the Institute for Community Inclusion at Children's Hospital Boston. During a fellowship in ethics at Harvard Medical School, he worked to develop a broad-based spiritual basis for bioethics. When he was at the Boston Medical Center, Dr. Coulter founded a group that explored the role of spirituality in pediatrics. His research focuses on issues faced by children with disabilities and their families who belong to various cultures. Dr. Coulter is active in the American Association on Mental Retardation and the Greater Boston Arc, and has been a consultant to the Massachusetts Department of Mental Retardation. He is co-editor of *The Theological Voice of Wolf Wolfensberger* (Haworth).

What gifts do people w/ disabilities bring to society?

How do they teach the rest of us to be human beings?

What is a human being?
What characteristics does a human being have?

Foreword

The history of the place of people with an intellectual disability in society has been characterised by a consistent denial of their "personhood" or "humaness." Even in the enlightened times of post modernism an intact intellect or mind is still the metric by which society judges the value of a person.

In many ways science has contributed to this phenomenon. Spectacular discoveries emerging from the human genome project have emphasized society's quest for the "perfect" child, born without imperfection of mind or body. Science is also breaking new barriers in the prevention or amelioration of disease leading to life expectancies earlier generations could only dream of.

In the field of scientific inquiry into the causes and "treatment" of intellectual disabilities we have made enormous advances in the last half of the century that have benefited people with disabilities and their families, especially in the western, industrialized world.

We have also been fortunate in having a parallel set of forces that have more philosophical foundations. Civil and human rights movements have assisted the emancipation of our brothers and sisters with a variety of disabilities.

However, there has been an uneasy relationship in this field between those who pursue a "scientific" approach and those who choose to emphasize the human rights approach. At the international level we have two organizations working to improve the quality of life of people with intellectual disabilities that symbolize the artificial divide between these two approaches. One is the International Association for the Scientific Study of Intellectual Disabilities (IASSID) and the other is the parent-based body, Inclusion International.

During my presidency of IASSID I have striven to achieve two goals. One has been a greater collaboration between scientists who approach

[Haworth co-indexing entry note]: "Foreword." Parmenter, Trevor R. Co-published simultaneously in *Journal of Religion, Disability & Health* (The Haworth Pastoral Press, an imprint of The Haworth Press, Inc.) Vol. 5, No. 2/3, 2001, pp. xix-xx; and: *Spirituality and Intellectual Disability: International Perspectives on the Effect of Culture and Religion on Healing Body, Mind, and Soul* (eds: William C. Gaventa, Jr. and David L. Coulter) The Haworth Pastoral Press, an imprint of The Haworth Press, Inc., 2001, pp. xiii-xiv. Single or multiple copies of this article are available for a fee from The Haworth Document Delivery Service [1-800-342-9678, 9:00 a.m. - 5:00 p.m. (EST). E-mail address: getinfo@haworthpressinc.com].

xiii

the question of "what is truth" from a variety of methodological and epistemological perspectives. This alone is a daunting task! The other goal has been to draw together the scientists and the very people they study into a stronger partnership.

The hallmark of science it is claimed, is its objectivity, but we have neglected over the years the very ingredient that identifies us as human beings–that is our subjective experiences, including our spirituality.

It was therefore a great joy to me personally, and I believe to the benefit of the 2000 Congress of IASSID, that we for the first time had dedicated sessions devoted to exploring this essential dimension of quality of life. It was even more gratifying that the organisers of this stream were able to include presentations from a variety of faiths.

I am hopeful that this initiative will blossom into a more permanent component of the work of IASSID through the formation of a Special Interest Research group. The exploration of the relationships between spiritual, physical and mental health will enrich our field. Hence this collection of papers for the Congress is a veritable harbinger for the continued growth of the Association.

Trevor R. Parmenter, PhD
President, IASSID
1996-2000

Preface

SPIRITUAL HEALTH AND PEOPLE WITH INTELLECTUAL DISABILITIES: INTERNATIONAL PERSPECTIVES AND INVITATIONS

In this volume, (co-published as a special double issue of *Journal of Religion, Disability & Health*), we are delighted to present a collection of articles on spirituality, religion, and people with intellectual disabilities which came from presentations at the 2000 Conference of the International Association for the Scientific Study of Intellectual Disabilities. These sessions were part of a first for the IASSID, an organized strand of sessions and papers focusing on the importance of spirituality and religion in supports and services for people with intellectual disabilities. Because this was a "first" for many of the presenters at an Association whose name focuses on the word "science" rather than "spirit," there was not a little uncertainty about how the topic and strand would be received. We should not have been worried. The welcome and hospitality was wonderful, as was the attendance at many of the sessions. Many said, "It is about time this was discussed."

Our goal for this strand was to have a series of international voices that could represent practitioners and researchers from major faith traditions and different parts of the world. The IASSID has done major position papers on aspects of physical health and psychological health for people with intellectual disabilities. Thus our organizing principle became the concept of "spiritual health," a framework for bridging the worlds of "science" and "faith," and exploring the ways that a variety of faith traditions, cultural backgrounds, and professional roles might help us move towards a consensus about what "spiritual health" means within specific cultures and faiths and across disciplines.

[Haworth co-indexing entry note]: "Preface." Gaventa, Bill, and David Coulter. Co-published simultaneously in *Journal of Religion, Disability & Health* (The Haworth Pastoral Press, an imprint of The Haworth Press, Inc.) Vol. 5, No. 2/3, 2001, pp. xxi-xxiv; and: *Spirituality and Intellectual Disability: International Perspectives on the Effect of Culture and Religion on Healing Body, Mind, and Soul* (eds: William C. Gaventa, Jr. and David L. Coulter) The Haworth Pastoral Press, an imprint of The Haworth Press, Inc., 2001, pp. xv-xviii. Single or multiple copies of this article are available for a fee from The Haworth Document Delivery Service [1-800-342-9678, 9:00 a.m. - 5:00 p.m. (EST). E-mail address: getinfo@haworthpressinc.com].

xv

We wanted papers that addressed the following issues:

1. How might "spiritual health" be defined from within a particular tradition and/or religious perspective?
2. What are traditions or themes from within those traditions that particularly relate to, or focus upon, persons with intellectual disabilities?
3. What are resources from within those traditions that can be drawn upon to enhance the lives of persons with intellectual disabilities and their families?
4. Outline and/or summarize creative initiatives (including practices, policies, and research) in parts of the world that draw upon those traditions to support people with intellectual disabilities and which attempt to integrate spiritual perspectives in human services and supports.

Our open invitation led to a series of papers that organized themselves into sessions on varied cultural and religious perspectives, theoretical perspectives, research, and creative models of ministry and practice. Some had been submitted to the conference without knowing about the Spiritual Health strand. A couple are from people who wanted to be present, but could not. We are very grateful to the authors, and to many who spent their own funds to come to Seattle. Some did much more. Chaplain Anja Vogelzang from the Netherlands produced a video of their model of worship for and with people with multiple disabilities as an accompaniment to her paper. We can't include it in this publication, but she has graciously made it available for order.

The international nature of the conference was underscored by the varied familiarity with English (the official language of the conference) expressed by the many speakers and participants. Some were quite fluent and others struggled to express themselves clearly. The universal language of spirituality and disability was heard through voices that reflected their country and culture of origin. The richness of this dialogue is preserved in the papers published here. As Editors, we have chosen to edit lightly in order to allow the reader to experience some of the atmosphere of the conference that brought together people from all over the world.

This volume of edited papers from the conference is simply a first step in addressing those questions and issues. There are so many voices that were not part of this first strand. We did not receive papers about Eastern or African religions, we would welcome those voices on this

Journal. We know there are many more models of creative research and practice around the world. The door and the dialogue are open. Here are some ways you can participate:

HELP FORM A SPECIAL INTEREST RESEARCH GROUP WITH IASSID

Become a founding member of the Special Interest Research Group of the IASSID that will become a network for dialogue and planning of future initiatives within this international association. You can represent any discipline or faith background. We need ten members of the IASSID to begin an official SIRG. The next conference is in Montpelier, France, in 2004. Membership in the IASSID is $75.00 per year, which includes a subscription to their *Journal of Intellectual Disability Research* ($50 without the journal.) Join by sending a check or money order made out "IASSID" to IASSID Membership Office, 31 Nottingham Way South, Clifton Park, NY 12065-1713.

If you want to be a member of the Special Interest Research Group on Spiritual Health, email that interest to Bill Gaventa, *gaventwi@umdnj.edu*, and indicate when you have joined the IASSID.

JOIN AN INTERNATIONAL LISTSERV ON SPIRITUALITY AND DISABILITY

Join an international listserv on Spirituality and Disability. Dr. John Swinton, at the University of Aberdeen in Scotland, is the founder of this listserv. It is a way of sharing ideas, resources and dialogue. To join the list serv, go to *http://<www.jiscmail.ac.uk/lists/disability-and-spirituality.html>*.

BECOME A REPRESENTATIVE FOR THIS JOURNAL WITHIN YOUR COUNTRY

As co-editors of the *Journal of Religion, Disability, & Health*, we are always looking for people who can represent our publication within their own country, and serve through our Editorial Advisory Board. Those representatives help recruit and review papers, encourage subscriptions, and develop awareness about JRDH. If you are interested, contact either Dr. David Coulter or Rev. Bill Gaventa.

Finally, we welcome your contribution of writing from your own research and practice. The questions which we posed on "spiritual health" are fully in line with the Vision statement we have for this Journal. They need much more careful exploration. They need "Guest Editors" who might take on a topic or question and organize an issue of the journal.

In Seattle, we were extremely grateful for those who responded to our invitation, and gratified by hospitality we received. As writer, speaker, and educator Parker Palmer points out, in the understandings of hospitality to the stranger within the major faith traditions, the gift is not really to the stranger, but to the host. As the hosts, thank you. We are now delighted to share with others the refined editions from our feast in Seattle, something much more than the "left-overs." We hope it whets your appetite for more.

Bill Gaventa, MDiv
David Coulter, MD

I. HEALING MIND, BODY, AND SOUL: THEORETICAL FOUNDATIONS FOR UNDERSTANDINGS OF SPIRITUAL HEALTH FOR PERSONS WITH INTELLECTUAL DISABILITIES

Recognition of Spirituality in Health Care: Personal and Universal Implications

David L. Coulter, MD

SUMMARY. Spirituality may be difficult to recognize among persons with significant intellectual and physical disabilities, yet it is present even when disability is so severe that consciousness is limited or absent. A clinical method is presented, based on the author's experience as a physician, that facilitates sharing of spirituality between caregivers and persons with disabilities. Caregivers must first accept their own spirituality and then seek to discover the spiritual essence of another person. Doing so provides insight into that which all persons have in common and leads (sometimes)

David L. Coulter is a member of the faculty with the Departments of Neurology, and Social Medicine, Harvard Medical School, Institute for Community Inclusion, Children's Hospital Boston, Boston, Massachusetts.

[Haworth co-indexing entry note]: "Recognition of Spirituality in Health Care: Personal and Universal Implications." Coulter, David L. Co-published simultaneously in *Journal of Religion, Disability & Health* (The Haworth Pastoral Press, an imprint of The Haworth Press, Inc.) Vol. 5, No. 2/3, 2001, pp. 1-11; and: *Spirituality and Intellectual Disability: International Perspectives on the Effect of Culture and Religion on Healing Body, Mind, and Soul* (eds: William C. Gaventa, Jr. and David L. Coulter) The Haworth Pastoral Press, an imprint of The Haworth Press, Inc., 2001, pp. 1-11. Single or multiple copies of this article are available for a fee from The Haworth Document Delivery Service [1-800-342-9678, 9:00 a.m. - 5:00 p.m. (EST). E-mail address: getinfo@haworthpressinc.com].

1

to a religious experience of the ground of all spirituality. The method has universal implications across levels of ability and disability, across cultures and world religions, and across value systems involving science, human service and politics. *[Article copies available for a fee from The Haworth Document Delivery Service: 1-800-342-9678. E-mail address: <getinfo@haworthpressinc.com> Website: <http://www.HaworthPress.com> © 2001 by The Haworth Press, Inc. All rights reserved.]*

KEYWORDS. Spirituality, caregiver, significant disability, clinical method, physician

SPIRITUALITY

Spirituality is an intensely personal and individual belief system usually not discoverable through reason alone. Spirituality can be expressed through statements of faith about the nature of one's identity, the impact of one's culture (including ethnicity, religious beliefs and healing practices), one's relationships of love and one's sense of meaning and purpose in life. It is easier to describe than define. We can recognize it in many diverse ways without ever really grasping "it" as an entity. Perhaps this is because spirituality is the essence of our subjective selfhood and thus resists objectification through definition. As subjective essence, it also cannot be partitioned or measured in relative terms. Thus we cannot say that a person's spirituality is less because he cannot express a sense of identity or purpose in life, because for him spirituality may consist in giving and receiving love or being part of a caring community.

Similarly, spirituality is not lessened because conscious expression is lessened (as for example following a severe brain injury). Consciousness may be a property of the brain, but spirituality is a property of the whole person (the subjective essence of being). This suggests that consciousness may not be required for spiritual personhood and spiritual essence or being could be present in a person who is no longer conscious. Spirituality does not disappear when we are asleep for the night, and I would argue that it also does not disappear just because a person will never wake up. Perhaps spiritual consciousness can be considered a mediation between the finitude of this world and the infinite aspect of being that transcends this world (Sulmasy, 1997). The absence of consciousness might then relieve the person from having to deal with the finite reality of the world and allow the person to exist solely in contemplation of the infinite. This is a fairly radical notion. If it is accepted, it leads to the conclusion that spirituality is present in every human being including those who are permanently unconscious or (neurologically speaking) in a persistent vegetative state.

Spirituality is different from a theory of mind in which one is able to represent oneself as different from someone else (an ability which is said to be lacking in some persons with intellectual disabilities) because spirituality comes from a deeper sense of awareness of one's self. Spirituality may be the awareness (conscious or not) upon which intelligence works to build a theory of mind. Howard Gardner, the author of the theory of multiple intelligences, considers and rejects the idea that spirituality is a type of intelligence (Gardner, 1999). Gardner's theory allows us to consider that persons with intellectual disabilities may have difficulty with certain types of intelligence, usually with what he calls linguistic, logico-mathematical and intrapersonal (theory of mind) intelligence. They may not have difficulty with other types of intelligence, such as musical, spatial, bodily-kinesthetic or interpersonal intelligence, however. If spirituality is not a kind of intelligence, then it is not linked to what is usually measured as IQ and can be richly present in persons with intellectual disabilities. Thus Gardner's theory validates what is common knowledge to all who minister with such persons.

With this understanding of spirituality, we might ask whether it is appropriate to do a "scientific study" of spirituality. The objective purposes and methods of science do not seem well suited to the study of spirituality. Yet we can study the objective correlates of spirituality with health or behavior, for example. We must avoid superficial correlations that seek to identify these objective correlates with the true subjective essence of spirituality, however. Perhaps it would be fair to say that scientific study of spirituality is acceptable as long as we also seek to understand spirituality in nonscientific terms.

Spirituality is present in all persons, from the most disabled to the most gifted, but may be hidden or blocked from the individual through denial or lack of reflection. It may also be hidden or blocked from others in a variety of ways. Sometimes the person does not want us to see it, and sometimes we do not want to see it and fail to look for it. In health care, it may be blocked by illness or disability that impedes caregivers from understanding the person's spiritual presence. One solution is to adopt a pastoral approach to clinical care in which the caregiver can "look three times" to experience the other person's spirituality (Coulter, 2001). These three looks will be familiar to those in pastoral care, but are much less apparent in clinical care and utilized all too rarely by health care providers.

To use this clinical method, the health care provider or caregiver must first examine his or her own spirituality. This can be done in a variety of ways (see for example Sulmasy, 1997). The three ways of looking described below will have little meaning for those who deny their own spirituality. Many health care providers choose not to take this first step of examining and accepting their own spirituality. For those who have taken this step, the three ways of looking will resonate with their own experience and enrich their personal and professional lives.

THREE WAYS OF LOOKING

The *first look* is to see the person as an individual human being, not just as a patient or as a clinical case but rather as a person with the "breath of life" of human consciousness. This can be harder than it sounds. We are so used to seeing people objectively through a variety of discernible characteristics (short, tall, fat, thin, young, old, pretty, ugly, graceful, awkward, smart, slow) that it is much more difficult to see them subjectively as individuals with the experience of being alive. This first look is an attempt to grasp the spiritual ground of the individual's existence. We can seek to know the answers to the questions, "Who is he?" "Where does he come from (what is his ethnicity or culture)?" "Who loves him and whom does he love (to whom does he belong)?" "What does he value in life (what is the meaning and purpose of his life)?" Answers to any of these questions can help us to understand his spirituality, but his spirituality is not limited or defined by these answers (or the questions).

What can we say about the person who is permanently unconscious, who is in a persistent vegetative state? What spirituality can we share with her? Perhaps we can glimpse an answer by visualizing the following scene, one that is surely familiar to many of us. An elderly woman with Alzheimer's disease is living in a nursing home, where she is confined to bed and does not recognize or interact with anyone around her. Although there are times when her eyes are open and she appears awake, she is not aware of anything or anyone and does not respond in a meaningful way. The doctors say she is in a persistent vegetative state and there is no reason to doubt that diagnosis. Next to her bed sits her husband of 60 years. He lives nearby, in the house where they raised their family, and comes to the nursing home every day to sit with his wife. He holds her hand, talks to her from time to time, and enjoys being with her whenever he can. The staff try to tell him that his wife is "no longer there" but he knows better. To him, she is most certainly still there and will be there as long as she is alive. The love that they shared for 60 years still holds them together, even if she can no longer respond to him. Is this love not a manifestation of their spirituality? And if the love they give to and receive from each other is present, is spirituality not still present for both of them?

Daniel Berrigan told the story of how he was working in a hospice for the "terminally ill" and would go every week to sit by the bed of a young boy who was totally incapacitated and could not communicate with others in any way. Like the elderly woman in the image above, the boy might be described as being in a persistent vegetative state. Berrigan said that he goes to try to hear what the young boy is saying in his silence and helplessness. Berrigan went on to say, "The way this young man lies in our world, silent and helpless, is the way God lies in our world. To hear what God is saying we must learn to hear what this young boy is saying" (Berrigan, 2000).

I too have sat by the bedside of a young patient who was in a persistent vegetative state, a girl I had known for several years as she lived with the severe disability that would ultimately take her life. In those final days just between Christmas and New Year's Day when the hospital was quiet and most patients were home with their families, I held her hand and talked to her about the good times she had had with her family and friends. I had no doubt she was still present and could sense that her subjective spiritual being was still evident in her mute, helpless state.

This first look is much like what Pellegrino and Thomasma call the virtue of compassion in clinical care, the ability to "suffer with" the patient and to understand the patient's experience of illness from his perspective. It is even closer to what they call empathy, the ability to feel and understand who the other person is (Pellegrino and Thomasma, 1993). Compassion and empathy are similar but are not the same as what we are seeking to achieve with this first look, however. They argue that compassion requires distance and objectivity, while this first look requires closeness and subjectivity if we are to see the person as a spiritual being.

This first look has its dangers. One of the dangers of subjectivity is an inability to see what is objectively best for the other person. This can limit one's effectiveness as a physician, for example. A young patient of mine was hospitalized recently for a severe life-threatening illness (a sudden shunt malfunction). I had known him since he was born 12 years earlier. I had fought to get the court order that treated his hydrocephalus at birth, and I had ensured he got therapy and services to overcome his disabilities during the years that followed. He was (and is) very close to me. Yet when he was recovering from this most recent illness, I realized that it was hard for me to remain objective about what he wanted and what was best for him. I came to rely on my colleagues to make the key clinical decisions about his treatment. This first look requires a clinician to remain aware of the different roles of physician and friend and to navigate carefully between them.

Another danger is to recognize the limits of compassion. Many years ago, I became very close to a young man whom I was treating for seizures (epilepsy). One day he called me while I was in clinic and we spoke for more than an hour. At first he was very distraught and crying, but by the end of our talk he seemed to feel better and we agreed to talk again soon. A short time later I got a call from a policeman who had come to his house because my patient had just committed suicide. They traced his phone calls and discovered that I was the last person to whom he had spoken. Many clinicians have had similar experiences and despite reassurances from friends and colleagues, we are still haunted by the feeling that perhaps we could have done more. With my awareness of his spirituality gleaned from this first look, I could connect with this young man but in the end I could not save his life. Perhaps I did all I could and perhaps he had called just to say goodbye. After all these years I still remember him fondly and sadly. To honor his memory, I shared his story so that others might learn from it and perhaps save the life of another young person in a similar situation (Coulter, 1980).

The *second look* is to see the person as a human being like myself. First we are aware of our own spirituality, what we know is central to our own existence as a person. Then we see that the other person has a spirituality like our own. From this awareness of our own spirituality, we seek to recognize in the other person that which we know to be central to our own existence. Knowing what it means to me to be alive, I can then try to realize what it means for the other person to be alive. I can say, "This is not just a person, this is a person just like myself." The purpose of this second look is to try to enter into the other person's point of view, to try to experience the other person's subjectivity, to try to appreciate what it means to the other person to be alive. Dunne has described this as a process of passing over from our standpoint into the other person's standpoint, and then returning to ourselves with a fresh awareness of what we share and a new awareness of what is essential in ourselves (Dunne, 1991). The first look showed us the person as a spiritual being; the second look shows us the spirituality that we have in common. With this second look, we can then value in the other person what we value most in ourselves. This is based on the shared awareness of our spirituality and is not based on the differences that may divide us. There are many types of differences that are used to define people, such as race, gender, ethnicity, sexual orientation, ability or disability. We can transcend those differences to see instead what binds us together in our spirituality. If I value in others what I value in myself, I now see that I must protect for others what I would protect for myself. What are these valuable things that warrant protection? Surely they must include the basic goods of life, liberty and happiness. Protecting life means a commitment to peace-making or pacifism, as well as opposition to death-making in all of its forms. Protecting liberty means a commitment to tolerance of differences and opposition to injustice based on those differences. Protecting happiness means a commitment to serving others through advocacy, direct action and community building and opposition to isolation and despair. Often we must confront our own learned attitudes toward differences and make peace with ourselves first before we can understand fully what this second look reveals and what it requires of us.

Bernard Wagner, as the President of the American Association on Mental Retardation, spoke of how he had come to see "the beauty and power of people with mental retardation" (Wagner, 2000). He did not mean this to be just a slogan or a patronizing view of being in an unequal relationship with another person. He meant it as a statement of belief that came from the heart and from his own experience of being with persons with intellectual disabilities. With this second look we can indeed come to see with our heart and soul the true beauty and power of people with intellectual disabilities. This experience of shared spirituality can lead to a love for the other person (Gourgey, 1999). Erich Fromm wrote, "If I can say, I love you, I must be able to say, I love in you everybody, I love through you the world, I love in you also myself" (Fromm, 1989). The second look is a way to experience this kind of love.

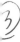

The *third look* is to see in the other person the ground of all being and all existence, the transcendence or divinity that informs our spirituality. With the third look we can say that we see in the other person the face of God. There are many ways to experience the face of God, as for example through poetry (DePree and DePree, 1974). Hauerwas wrote, "God's face is the face of the retarded" (Hauerwas, 1986), and with this third look we can see the face of God in the face of persons with disabilities with whom we interact. But the first two ways of looking may be necessary before we can achieve this third look. Spirituality includes our relationship with God, but it may equally be God's relationship with us. When we share our spirituality with another and experience that person's spirituality as valuable as our own, we share that relationship as well. In doing so, we participate in the source of all spirituality which is surely a reflection of God. The sense of this is like that in 1 John 4:16, "God is love, and anyone who live in love lives in God, and God lives in him."

My spiritual journey has at times been troubled and it has been hard for me sometimes as a physician to find God in church (Coulter, 1991). Perhaps for this reason I have sought to find God through love and service to others, as John teaches (1 John 4:16). Through many encounters with patients during my 27 years as a physician, I came to see and understand the three ways of looking outlined here. I have experienced the third look on only a few occasions, but those moments have been truly life-changing.

One of the most memorable experiences of this third look occurred while I was visiting a state-operated residential center for persons with mental retardation. I was there as an expert consultant for the United States Department of Justice, which had sued the state alleging that the care being provided did not meet the constitutional standard for health and safety. I was shadowed by lawyers for both sides and the atmosphere was certainly contentious. One of my tasks was to meet and evaluate the care provided to a selected group of individuals residing there. We entered one building where approximately 40 residents were lying on mats on the floor. I sought out the person I had come to meet and found him lying there, unable to speak or move. I knelt down, held his hand and spoke to him for a while. He opened his eyes and looked at me as I talked to him, and in that moment I knew immediately that we were experiencing this third look. I cannot explain how or why it happened, or why it happened with him and not with any of the other residents I met on that tour. But it did happen and I was changed by the experience.

Kleinert described his own experience of the third look in a brief encounter with a young student with profound disabilities whom he was trying (with great difficulty) to teach the 25 steps of toothbrushing. At one point the student suddenly looked deeply into the teacher's eyes and Kleinert saw "a flash of insight into all that life was about, a glimpse into a personhood far deeper and more communicative than all our measures of intellectual capacity, of human wit and skill." It was for him an

experience of the face of God. Kleinert adds, "Perhaps at the very moment in which we are laid most bare in the eyes of another (even if that
other is a person with profound mental retardation), God has his best
chance of getting to us" (Kleinert, 2001).

The first two looks can be experienced with many persons, once we
make the effort. But the third look seems to be very uncommon and comes when we least expect it. It may happen only once or twice in our
lives. Perhaps this is because it comes to us when God is ready to show
us His presence, and we cannot determine or control God's grace. Although I have suggested that we see the face of God in this third look, it
may be presumptuous to think that we can truly see His face. Like Moses in Exodus 33: 18-23, we can hope to see God's splendor reflected in
the eyes of another person, and that is enough for a lifetime.

UNIVERSAL IMPLICATIONS

The three ways of looking can be applied in ways that transcend the
boundaries that divide us. They can be applied across the spectrum of
ability and disability, as was shown in the examples above. It is easy
enough to recognize and share the experience of spirituality with people
who are most like us. It is more difficult to do so with people who are
different because of the presence of intellectual or physical disabilities,
but it can be done. Spirituality is not linked to intelligence and can be
discovered among individuals with disabilities if we open ourselves up
to them. I have argued that the spiritual essence of being persists even in
the absence of consciousness and shared several stories that support this
argument. Some would disagree and argue that consciousness is required for what is called personhood or membership in the human community. Those who do so usually do not recognize or value the role of
spirituality in human existence, however. If we do not share this basic
presupposition, we cannot expect to convince each other. If spirituality
is recognized and valued as an aspect of human existence, then it must
be present in all persons regardless of their ability or disability. When
we understand the difference between consciousness and spirituality as
described above, we see how spiritual presence transcends literally all
of the boundaries of ability and disability. Recognizing spirituality
through application of the three ways of looking permits a universal affirmation of the value and worth of all persons. This affirmation carries
with it a commitment to protect the life, liberty and happiness of all persons as well.

The three ways of looking are relevant across all *cultures and religions* as well. Spirituality is found in answers to questions about one's identity, cultural and ethnic background, relationships of love, and beliefs about the meaning and purpose of life. These are surely universal questions that are present in all cultures and religions. With the first look we seek to understand the other person's spirituality as she experiences it from her own cultural and religious background, through learning what her answers might be to these universal questions. With the second look we share our own spirituality and seek to find the common ground that links us together as spiritual beings. The second look conveys the admonition to love your neighbor as yourself, which is often called the Universal Rule because of it's presence in most cultures and religions. Rabbi Hillel wrote (from a Jewish perspective), "Love your neighbor as yourself. All the rest is commentary. Go now and learn." The meaning of the third look would likely vary across cultures and religions, and the experience of the third look may be too rare to permit easy generalizations. I expect that individuals in many cultures and religions have had the experience described in this third look, once they have lived with others in the ways suggested by the first two looks. Sharing these experiences of the source or ground of all spirituality as it is understood in each particular culture or religion would likely help us to see that this too is universal.

The three ways of looking also convey significant implications across *value systems*. Human-centered systems that value individuals can recognize the spiritual uniqueness of all persons. This would lead to universal welcoming and inclusion of people with disabilities in social, cultural and religious communities. The second look in particular leads to a commitment to protecting the life, liberty and happiness of all persons, regardless of the differences that may divide us. Theories of justice based on this recognition of the universal value and worth of all persons lead to political systems that emphasize peace-making instead of death-making. Scientific value systems can learn from the three ways of looking how to appreciate the value of individual differences. One of the dangers of modern science and genetics is the cult of perfection which seeks to eliminate these differences and to promote a single standard of health and well-being. With the three looks we can learn to see the uniqueness of each individual as well as the universal spirituality that binds us all to each other. Science and genetics can recognize the adaptive and evolutionary significance of individual differences and replace the cult of perfection with respect for human diversity.

Recognizing spirituality in health care is a challenge for all care-givers. The first step is to accept the role of spirituality in our own lives. With the three ways of looking we can then learn to appreciate the spirituality of others, particularly those with intellectual and physical disabilities. This personal recognition leads to universal implications that affect health care delivery, transcultural understanding and social, political and scientific systems that value persons with disabilities. My hope is that this simple clinical technique could result in changes that would enrich all of us and improve our world.

REFERENCES

Berrigan, B. (Spring, 2000). God is love. *Noah Homes Newsletter* (Spring Valley, CA), p. 2.

Coulter, D.L. (1980). The unfairness of life for children with handicaps. *Journal of the American Medical Association*, 244, 1207-1208.

Coulter, D.L. (1991). A pushed-away Catholic. *Notre Dame Magazine*, 20 (1), 78-79.

Coulter, D.L. (2001). Three ways of looking: A pastoral approach to clinical care (Editorial). *Journal of Religion, Disability and Health*, 4 (4), 1-5.

DePree, G., DePree, G. (1974). *Faces of God*. New York: Harper and Row.

Dunne, J.S. (1991). *The peace of the present: An unviolent way of life*. Notre Dame, IN: University of Notre Dame Press.

Fromm, E. (1989). *The art of loving*. New York City, NY: Harper Collins.

Gardner, H. (1999). *Intelligence reframed.* New York City, NY: Basic Books.

Gourgey, C. (1999). Love-and its absence-in the caregiving relationship. *Journal of Religion, Disability and Health*, 3 (4), 57-72.

Kleinert, H.L. (2001). The three looks: The persons we profess to teach. *Journal of Religion, Disability and Health*, 4 (4), 77-90.

Pellegrino, E.D. & Thomasma, D.C. (1993). *The virtues in medical practice*. New York City, NY: Oxford University Press.

Sulmasy, D.P. (1997). *The healer's calling: A spirituality for physicians and other health care professionals*. New York: Paulist Press.

Wagner, B. (2000). Presidential address: Changing visions into reality (Unpublished paper): *American Association on Mental Retardation*.

Authenticity in Community: Theory and Practice of an Inclusive Anthropology in Care for Persons with Intellectual Disabilities

Herman P. Meininger, PhD

SUMMARY. Care and support for persons with intellectual disabilities are based upon a normative anthropology, an image of man which structures professional care practices. The normative anthropology of contemporary care practices is closely related to the dominating concept of the autonomous individual. The concept of the autonomous individual–as well as its relational alternative–has an exclusive character and is derived from an intellectualistic and substantialist interpretation of being human. Therefore, this concept cannot serve as a moral ground for care for persons with intellectual disabilities. Although sources of this interpretation can be found in mainstream western theological and philosophical traditions, in early and in modern Christian theological traditions,

Herman P. Meininger served for nearly twenty years as a chaplain in a service organization for persons with intellectual disabilities. He is Senior Research Fellow to the Willem van den Bergh Chair for Ethics and Care for Persons with Intellectual Disabilities at the Department of Theology of the Vrije Universiteit, Amsterdam, The Netherlands.

Address correspondence to: Dr. H.P. Meininger, Department of Theology, Vrije Universiteit, De Boelelaan 1105, 1081 HV Amsterdam, The Netherlands (E-mail: H.P. Meininger@th.vu.nl).

[Haworth co-indexing entry note]: "Authenticity in Community: Theory and Practice of an Inclusive Anthropology in Care for Persons with Intellectual Disabilities." Meininger, Herman P. Co-published simultaneously in *Journal of Religion, Disability & Health* (The Haworth Pastoral Press, an imprint of The Haworth Press, Inc.) Vol. 5, No. 2/3, 2001, pp. 13-28; and: *Spirituality and Intellectual Disability: International Perspectives on the Effect of Culture and Religion on Healing Body, Mind, and Soul* (eds: William C. Gaventa, Jr. and David L. Coulter) The Haworth Pastoral Press, an imprint of The Haworth Press, Inc., 2001, pp. 13-28. Single or multiple copies of this article are available for a fee from The Haworth Document Delivery Service [1-800-342-9678, 9:00 a.m. - 5:00 p.m. (EST). E-mail address: getinfo@haworth pressinc.com].

13

traces can also be found of an 'inclusive anthropology.' This inclusive anthropology offers important clues for a moral view of care and support for persons with intellectual disabilities. In this normative framework the emphasis is on authenticity and community. As a consequence, care and support for persons with intellectual disabilities are considered to be processes of continuing interpretation in which the development of particular virtues, skills and attitudes of professional caregivers plays a decisive role. *[Article copies available for a fee from The Haworth Document Delivery Service: 1-800-342-9678. E-mail address: <getinfo@haworthpressinc.com> Website: <http://www.HaworthPress.com>* © *2001 by The Haworth Press, Inc. All rights reserved.]*

KEYWORDS. Ethics, theology, anthropology, intellectual disability, caring relationships

RELEVANCE OF PHILOSOPHICAL ANTHROPOLOGY FOR CARE FOR PERSONS WITH INTELLECTUAL DISABILITIES

Some years ago, Mattijn Mataheru, who works as a special educator in a Dutch residential service organization, wrote a dissertation on early recognition of behavioral disorders in persons with intellectual disabilities. He describes the difficult and often toilsome processes of caregivers who try to form an understanding of a well-balanced image of their care-recipients and strive to set adequate objectives of care. His research clearly demonstrates that the essence of these processes can only be fully understood within the framework of the normative-anthropological and normative-ethical views of the caregivers. Caregivers often have many false or negative images of persons with intellectual disabilities. Objectives of care are usually not formulated from the perspective of the care recipient. A clear image of the individual with intellectual disabilities is absent in many cases or it is limited to the content of medical and psychological diagnostic records. Mataheru considers this lack of conscious and careful image-making to be an important cause of many behavioral problems and many other 'persistent problems in care' (Mataheru, 1995, pp. 34-36).

This observation points at two fundamental dimensions of care which are not often expressed in this way (see Siegenthaler 1983, 1993; Bleidick, 1990). First, images of individual human beings and objectives of care are basic elements of what I would call the 'structuring perspective' of care. This 'structuring perspective' of care is a fundamental dimension of care because images and objectives serve as an ultimate referential framework for the caregiver's motivation, attitude and practice. Secondly, these images and objectives have their roots in the more or less coherent relation between the image the caregiver has of the care recipient on the one hand, and the self image of the caregiver on the other hand. 'Structuring perspectives' of care are easily recognized in the various approaches of care for and contact with persons who have intellectual disabilities. Also, scientific definitions and paradigmatic conceptualizations of intellectual disability are expressions of a 'structuring perspective' of care. Of course, these approaches, definitions and conceptualizations can only be understood within the context of historical and socio-cultural circumstances. In their plurality, they may be seen as expressions of views of being human and views of 'the good life.' This means that ultimately every 'structuring perspective,' every web of images of the other, all self-images and objectives in life, and objectives in care have roots in a normative anthropology, a moral ideal of being human (Meininger, 1998, pp. 43-74, passim).

Now, an important question arises. Can a 'structuring perspective' and its implicit normative anthropology be judged? Is there a viewpoint, an ultimate standard, from which the plurality of concepts of 'being human' and 'being good' can be evaluated? Or, are there as many views as there are normative concepts of being human? Or, is it irrelevant to raise this question, as some 'postmodern' philosophers have claimed? In this article I cannot go deeper into the problems evoked by this question, but at least it has to be mentioned, because my position must be seen within the framework of this problem. This position is that normative judgments about images of being human and about objectives in care are not only possible, but also can be accounted for.

The first argument for this position is that it is very possible to develop a normative anthropology within the framework of a religious or philosophical tradition and to evaluate this anthropology on the basis of its own internal criteria. A second argument is that external criteria may also be used for this evaluation. For instance: a normative anthropology can be tested by asking the question of whether all human beings are really included in it. Put differently: is the existence of persons with (severe) intellectual disabilities a challenge to its universal validity? Only such an 'inclusive anthropology' can be an unambiguous basis for the practice of caring for persons with intellectual disabilities. Only on the basis of an 'inclusive anthropology' can this care be seen as meaningful human action.

So the question is how the 'structuring perspective' of contemporary care can be evaluated on the basis of the external criterion, whether it–consciously or unconsciously–excludes or includes certain persons. An analysis of this contemporary normative anthropology could reveal whether it actually is 'inclusive,' in the sense that it does not exclude persons with (severe) intellectual disabilities. If that is the case, then it can claim to have basic relevance for a normative ethics and for a humane practice of care. If not, then the time has come to do the groundwork for the development of a different normative anthropology.

DOMINANCE OF THE IMAGE
OF THE AUTONOMOUS INDIVIDUAL

The dominant image of man in contemporary western society is also the dominant image of man in care for persons with intellectual disabilities. It is the image of the free, independent citizen, equipped with individual and social rights, who assertively stands up for his interests as an individual and who is self-determined and responsible. This citizen expects from the society in which he lives nothing but the continuous production of a maximal offer of free choice. That would enable his self-realization according to his own scheme or project. Most documents published by official bodies, organized interest groups of parents and organizations for care and support of persons with intellectual disabilities support this ideal of the autonomous individual. Also 'spiritual health' of 'quality of life' are measured by standards of autonomy and subsequent intentional action. New laws in several European countries clearly express the fact that individual autonomy is considered to be the central moral value in health care. This value protects the individual against unwanted interventions of others. Moreover it makes it mandatory for others to respect the individual perspective of any fellow human being, the 'life from the inside,' regardless of the views of these others on 'being human' or 'the good life' (Reinders, 1996, pp. 5-8).

Transferred from the sphere of political philosophy, autonomy refers to a mere individual pattern of value, a sovereign subjectivity, which can effectively be protected by law. This autonomy is the means to and the ultimate aim and ideal of human development away from dependence into independence. Its project is emancipation and escape from tutelage and unwanted interference by all others. The task of the self, the autonomous subject, consists in a continuous breaking away from human interactions manifesting themselves as unequal power relationships. In this frame of reference the fellow human being is emphatically seen as a potential opponent of one's own process of self-realization. The other person represents the danger of heteronomy and of violation of territory. Therefore, it seems necessary to create circumstances in which individuals are secured against unwanted interference by way of negotiations, contracts, and laws.

The Canadian philosopher, Charles Taylor, has argued that this concept of autonomy contains a valuable and powerful ideal (Taylor, 1991, p. 26). This ideal demonstrates the existence of a well-determined and unique way of being human, that is *mine*. Taylor speaks of the ideal of authenticity. Authenticity means: being faithful to oneself, being faithful to that form of human existence that, I, in my life have gradually become to recognize as mine. But this ideal of authenticity has developed into a concept of autonomy that contains many problems. Taylor particularly mentions the subjectivity, the moral relativism and the complacency which seem to be part and parcel of this concept. He ultimately rejects the dominant concept of individual autonomy and considers it to be a degeneration of the moral ideal of authenticity, in which human life is seen as having fundamentally a dialogical character (Taylor, 1991, p. 33).

Even though I agree with Taylor's criticism of the ideal of individual autonomy, my own criticism has its starting point in the inclusiveness/exclusiveness of the dominant concept of autonomy. Does this concept include persons who are not or only partially capable of speaking for themselves, who have been or will never be capable of doing so? I believe it does not. The political-philosophical interest that is manifest in the image of the autonomous individual, makes invisible two important and inevitable facts. Firstly, the actual dependence of persons with intellectual disabilities cannot be eliminated by social or legal measures. Rights of patients can stop abuse of unequal power relationships, but they cannot neutralize the state of dependence. Secondly, this dependence necessitates a relationship of care and support that originates from a moral engagement which cannot be reduced to economical and legal relationships (Reinders, 1996, p. 15). At the level of anthropology this means that the image of the autonomous individual fails in confrontation with persons with severe intellectual disabilities. It breaks down when applied to those persons whose lack of individual autonomy, in the abovementioned sense, is a major characteristic of their life.

It is often said that persons with intellectual disabilities should live 'as autonomously as possible' or 'as normally as possible' or 'as much included in the community as possible.' This way of putting things clearly exposes a normative anthropology that, in confrontation with persons with severe intellectual disabilities, sees itself more and more pushed back. Eventually, this anthropology cannot explain in a positive sense that the value of life with intellectual disabilities–or even human life in general–can be based on other human characteristics than the ones that are highly appreciated within the framework of the dominant concept of individual autonomy (Edwards, 1997).

SOURCES AND ALTERNATIVES OF THE CONCEPT OF INDIVIDUAL AUTONOMY

For some readers, it may come as a surprise that, for an explanation of the origins of the concept of individual autonomy, I do not refer to great philosophers of the Age of Reason, like Descartes or Kant. The reason is that the sources of contemporary concepts of individual autonomy can be found much earlier in history. Of course, it cannot be denied that the philosophy of the Enlightenment has a major influence on the self-image of modern man. But even these philosophers presume the existence of a human 'self,' of personal identity. This self can be found by introspection into the inner life. This introspection leads to an understanding of oneself. Charles Taylor describes this process as a 'radical reflexivity' leading to the discovery of the 'first person point of view' which is the normative nucleus of human existence. Taylor attributes this discovery to the Church Father Augustine (Reinders, 1995, p. 22; Horne, 1991).

Some aspects of Augustine's anthropology, which are important for the continuation of my argument, will be explained. Crucial in this anthropology is its basis in the belief that man is made in the image of God and that God in whose image man is made is the Trinitarian God of Christian faith. This means that mankind reflects in a certain way this Trinity. To express this threefold nature of being human, Augustine uses the concepts of *memoria, intellectus* and *voluntas,* in another context also *mens, notitia sui* and *amor sui.* There is another important aspect of Augustine's anthropology: as he understood the Trinity as an internal relationship of the Divine self to itself, he also understood the human person as a being that is primarily related to itself. The self-relationship within the divine Trinity is reflected and represented in the rational and reflective capacities of the human soul. This relationship of the self to the self precedes any external relationships (Meininger, 1998, pp. 161-162). Put briefly, Augustine describes man as a sustance that is enclosed in itself. This substance can only be known by the actualization and expression of potential capacities and the qualities that characterize this substance. In relation to this characterization of man all human relationships are of secondary nature. They are derivatives of the original self-relationship. This foundational anthropological position returns in the Age of Reason in the form of the concept of autonomy and the modern concept of the individual person. It is an anthropology in which self-consciousness and rational self-determination on the basis of one's inner life is the supreme good.

It is not difficult to see that this intellectualist and reflective view of being human has a tendency of exclusiveness. The most important exclusion is not only based on the disproportionate emphasis on intellect and reflexivity as exclusive human characteristics. It may also be found in the negation of the constitutive meaning of human relationships for being human. It is exactly the phenomenon of human relationship which both in philosophy and theology has become the major starting point for the criticism of this anthropology (MacMurray, 1961). In this criticism can be found the first traces of an 'inclusive anthropology.'

Limiting myself to contemporary theological reflections, I would like to draw attention to one of the famous theologians from Tübingen, Germany, Jürgen Moltmann. He has tried to develop a 'social Trinitarian doctrine' as opposed to Augustine's 'psychological Trinitarian doctrine' (Moltman, 1980, 1991, 1993). In Augustine's theology and anthropology Moltmann distinguishes two central problems. The first has already been explained: the description of the substance of God and of man is focused on internal relationships. Secondly, these internal relationships have a 'monarchial' structure: the Father stands above the Son and the Spirit and, thus, in human beings soul stands above body and man above woman. Moltmann calls this an 'anthropology of dominion' (Moltmann, 1993, pp. 241, 244). Moltmann then proposes a new definition of divine (and human) Trinity as 'a community in which persons are not defined by power or possessions, but by their relations to and with one another' (Moltmann, 1980, p. 215). 'Community' cannot exist without openness to others. Community exists as a durable invitation and exhortation to communion. This openness also implies openness to the future, to the deepening, enrichment and fulfillment of relationships. So the essence of divine and human being cannot be comprehended in the static categories of a classical doctrine of being, but only in the categories of a dynamic historical relationship. For Moltmann, being human means living in a relationship which stands open to the eschatological destination of man. Rather than individual autonomy, "sociality" (community in the same space and time) and "generativity" (community of generations through time) are keywords in his description of being human.

However, Moltmann's relational description of being human does not answer some important questions. For instance, he has not paid any attention to the authenticity of the individual. Although I do not want to slip back into a postmodernist individualism, in care and support for persons with intellectual disabilities, I want to hold on to the ideal of authenticity as formulated by Charles Taylor. Furthermore, it should be seen that relationships between God and man, and among human beings are continuously denoted by Moltmann in static ontological categories. Human language, his 'reflective-responsive existence' remain important presuppositions for the possibility of human communion and community. Thus, also this relational conceptualization of being human cannot unambiguously be considered as an inclusive anthropology. In the struggle between *relatio* and *substantia,* the latter seems to be predominant, because it serves as an indispensable presupposition. Traces of thinking in terms of substantiality and subjectivity are clearly present in Moltmann's alternative of the image of man as an autonomous individual and these traces disturb the development of a real inclusive anthropology. If the authenticity of a person cannot be described in categories as reflexivity, rationality or discursive language, does this mean that this person is excluded from human communion? Can such a being be seen as a human person? Can such a being have anything like a personal identity at all? The answers to these questions have decisive significance for the moral practice of caring for and support of persons with intellectual disabilities.

AUTHENTICITY IN COMMUNITY:
THE SEARCH FOR AN INCLUSIVE ANTHROPOLOGY

It may be clear that an inclusive anthropology cannot define being human as a neutral substance, which develops into a subject or a moral being by using of some accidental characteristics or qualities. Even in the context of a social anthropology, such an image of being human gives space to the exclusion of some human beings from being human persons. Two authors, the Greek-Orthodox theologian John Zizioulas and the Canadian protestant theologian Douglas John Hall, designed–both from their own particular perspective–a radical inclusive anthropology. In this contribution, I especially refer to Zizioulas because, as Moltmann, he mainly draws from sources in early Christian Trinitarian theology. However, he turns to three contemporaries of Augustine who are known as the Cappadocian Fathers: Basil of Cesarea, Gregory of Nyssa and Gregory of Nazianzus.

Zizioulas does not consider the personal being of God and man as a static entity that is closed in itself, but as 'ek-stasis of being.' This *ekstasis* is a movement toward a community of persons; it aims at affirmation of the other. God only exists as free movement toward community. But at the same time this movement toward community is unique and unrepeatable, it is also *hypostasis*. Any movement toward community has its own recognizable identity. "Without these two conditions, being falls into an a-personal reality, defined and described like a mere 'substance,' i.e., it becomes an a-personal thing" (Zizioulas, 1975, p. 408). Community, freedom and love (ekstasis) make a particular personal being (hypostasis) to a 'self.' Vigorously, Zizioulas states that community, freedom and love are constitutive for the mere existence of this being. As God is freedom and love, being human is freedom and love. The divine Trinity serves as a model for this type of being. Trinity is a community in which one person is constituted by the other. The one receives his existence from the hand of the other. God does not exist in *what* He is for others, but in *who* He is for a particular other. Father, Son and Holy Spirit are not roles or modalities of a particular entity, but names that refer to specific relationships. As man has been created in the image of God, being human exists in the form of a community in which persons receive from each other their unique identities, each from the hand of the other. Human persons do not exist in *what* they are for each other, not in their intellectual capacities or influencing powers, but in *who* they are for each other.

So, here we find an anthropology in which substance and relation are not two separate elements. Also, relation is not a secondary attribute of substance. On the contrary, the relational perspective is all-embracing. The authenticity of a human being cannot be deducted from an underlying, universal, abstract and undetermined general being of which it is an accidental expression. It exclusively exists and is knowable in a distinct and concrete relationship. I do not primarily exist as a specimen of the human species, but as Herman. And I can only be Herman because others, for whom I am the other, call me Herman. Being a person consists in the freedom to be 'other.' Being different in terms of characteristics and qualities is not constitutive for being a person, being 'the other' is.

In the framework of this inclusive anthropology, relations between persons with intellectual disabilities and their family-members and professional caregivers neither depend on the presence or absence of certain natural capacities or abilities nor on the potential of improvement. The limitations of persons who have intellectual disabilities lose their constitutive significance if and when others are oriented towards the unique authenticity of the other. Many of us may have experienced encounters with persons with disabilities in which disabilities are present, but at the same time they become transparent and are in a sense invisible and irrelevant. The reason is that it is an encounter of John and Andy, of Rupert and Anna. It is an encounter of persons with a name that marks their own unique life story embedded in a web of relations. This experience reveals the normative character of an inclusive anthropology. It has basic importance for the 'structuring perspective' of care and support, its orienting images and objectives. The sketched inclusive anthropology gives room to a fully and equally valued position of persons with disabilities because it does not measure their existence by standards of self-consciousness, language skills or rational reflexivity. It aims at a relationship between caregivers and care recipients in which the *who* of the other precedes the *what*. In such an anthropology, the authenticity of a person is not the result of a particular arrangement of empirical facts, characteristics or qualities, but a gift that may be expected from the other in reciprocity. Douglas John Hall remarks: "The I.Q. test does not disclose the essence of the human any more than does the accumulation of deeds and achievements ('good works') that are products of an active and perhaps aggressive will. . . . We have been conditioned to locate the essence of *Homo sapiens* (as the nomenclature itself testifies) in rationality, freedom, spirituality, consciousness, moral sensibility, memory, and many other qualities of being. The relational conception of the *imago,* resting on the presupposition that being itself is relational, insists that all of these endowments are only secondary considerations—means, not ends. They are means, namely, to the end that we may be able to enter into the rather complex relationships for which we are intended" (Hall, 1986, pp. 115-116).

Of course, Zizioulas knows that in this world such a community can only be found in a imperfect and incomplete form. Theologically spoken, this imperfection is caused by human sinfulness. The movement toward community, therefore, often perverts into a movement toward division and opposition. Authenticity perverts into individualism and enmity. Under these circumstances community becomes limited to an 'arrangement of peaceful coexistence' which lasts as long as it serves the interests of the parties involved (Zizioulas, 1994, p. 10). Then, the other human being is not any more the one from whose hand I receive my existence, but he is–as for instance with Sartre–the ultimate threat to my existence. Difference between persons, the otherness of others, is not the result of a movement toward community, but its motivating force. However, difference may come into the possession of a 'individual rational actor' who keeps unlimited control of this possession by defining scales by which the other has to be measured and judged. Then, knowing the other is not any more a matter of love, but a matter of individualizing, fragmentizing and anatomizing, as it is common in the framework of a static-ontological view of being human. In Zizioulas' words: "Difference becomes division, and persons become individuals" (Zizioulas, 1975, p. 425). In Douglas John Hall's reflections on man as *imago Dei* (Hall, 1986, p. 128) a similar distinction has been made between essential, authentic humanity and existential, inauthentic humanity. Essential humanity is defined as a 'being-with' (coexistence), which implicates a being-for (pro-existence) and a being-together (communion, community, covenant). Existential humanity is defined as a 'being-alone' (autonomy), which implicates a being-against (estrangement), and a being-above (attempt at mastery) or a being-below (escape from responsibility). In an inclusive anthropology all human persons are seen in the perspective of 'being-with.' This is the only perspective from which care for persons with severe intellectual disabilities can be seen as a meaningful human activity.

PRACTICAL–ETHICAL IMPLICATIONS OF AN INCLUSIVE ANTHROPOLOGY

My first step has been to explain that any 'structuring perspective' (orienting images and objectives in care and support) is based upon a normative anthropology. Furthermore, I have explained that only an anthropology that has its ontological starting point in the principle of authenticity in community can unambiguously include persons with intellectual disabilities. Such an anthropology is able to avoid the danger inherent to care relationships to play the individual off against the collective, the subject against the object, the *what* against the *who*. Now, finally, the question presents itself of what the practical consequences of this argument might be.

To answer this question, we have to remember that in an inclusive anthropology there is a close connection between our image of the other and our self-image. The question 'who is the other?' immediately leads to the question 'who am I?' and answers to these questions always are interdependent. In care and support a basic question for caregivers is the question 'how do I see the other?' Care and support thus can be described as interpretative activities. The authenticity of the persons involved in the relationship of caring relationships is constantly interpreted. Caregivers are challenged to discover the authenticity of care receivers again and again. This is an activity in which the authenticity of the caregiver is fully involved.

That is why 'hermeneutical competence' can be seen as the basic professional skill of caregivers (Reinders, 1996, p. 37), 'imaginative anticipation' as the characterizing moral attitude an *subtilitas* (subtlety) as the basic virtue of professional caregivers (Clegg, 2000). I will shortly elaborate upon these concepts.

Skills–'Hermeneutical Competence'

What does it mean to interpret the other (with or without intellectual disabilities) with respect for his or her authenticity? This is the central moral question regarding hermeneutical competence. I mention some important aspects.

First of all, it is important to be aware of one's particular position as an observer. Observing the other does not consist in a division between a subject and an object and a corresponding objectifying of the other, but in an engagement. To observe someone is to be in relation with him or her. The way in which we relate to others is always influenced by our convictions and by our ideals about meaningful human life. Therefore, the position of an observer always implies in a certain way 'being touched' (Kleinbach 1994, p. 186). There is no neutral position of 'imagelessness' ('Bildlosigkeit,' Bleidick 1992, p. 106), no 'view from nowhere.' Interpretation means engagement, means movement toward communion. Neutral, merely descriptive, value-free accounts do not exist. Any interpretation leads to a particular attitude and sometimes to particular acts. This attitude and these acts have to be tested by the norm of respect for the authenticity of the other (Meininger 1996).

A second moral aspect in connection with hermeneutical competence is the circumstance that there are several potential positions of observance, several modalities of 'being touched.' Interpreting, then, ideally is a communal process consisting in a dialogue of competing perspectives and interpretations. I am not the only observer–there are parents, brothers and sisters, friends, colleagues whose interpretations have to be reflected upon in order to approximate a well-balanced image. Because, time after time, and person after person, new encounters are possible, because every new encounter leads to new experiences, interpretation is a never-ending activity. This activity demands from caregivers a great openness for others, for new experiences in the future and for a variety of interpretations.

Thirdly, hermeneutic competence presupposes self-criticism. To interpret the other is to interpret the other's authenticity in the context of a shared community. Therefore, this interpretation is at the same time a form of self-interpretation. Any statement about the other implies a statement about my self-image and about the image of those who I consider to be my peers. Psychologically, this implies that projections of my own inhibitions and ideals are always present. If they weren't present, I wasn't there. But at the same time they have to be articulated, analyzed and criticized in order to prevent them from disturbing an open encounter with the other. This not only pertains to the individual projections of the persons involved but also to the projection of collective ideals and prejudices which are a part of our culture. The interpreting community surrounding a person who has intellectual disabilities should be aware of the destructive influence such ideals and prejudices may have on the emergence of the authenticity of the other and of oneself.

Fourthly, these processes of interpretation and the provisional results of these processes basically have an ethical character. They contain presumptions about the good life and about human destination. Therefore a 'dialogue of moral frameworks' (Schwöbel, 1989, p. 137) should be a key element in any hermeneutical course of action. Hermeneutical competence includes the ability to enter into the heart of moral intuitions and convictions.

Attitude–'Imaginative Anticipation'

Some years ago, I introduced the concept of 'imaginative anticipation' as a moral attitude that may be considered as the ethical implication of an inclusive anthropology (Meininger, 1998). This attitude is characterized by anticipation because authenticity in community cannot be fully experienced and all the same it serves as an orienting image for human relations in care and support. This attitude also has an imaginative character, because it does not anticipate something already known, but the fulfillment of a promise. In Christian faith and in Christian theology this fulfillment is the central theme of eschatology. In the Bible, eschatological fulfillment is pictured in a great variety of metaphorical expressions and stories which evoke and inspire faith and theological reflection. I think the hopeful and perseverant expectation that is indispensable in relating to others–especially relating to persons with severe intellectual disabilities–can also be tracked down in the utopian images of other religions and philosophies of life. Wolfgang Jantzen for instance considers the 'loss of the ability to imagine a new utopia' to be the greatest threat to humane care and support for persons with intellectual disabilities (Jantzen, 1991).

Virtue–'Subtlety'

From the above it may be clear why I have introduced *subtilitas* as the key virtue of caregivers (Meininger, 1998, p. 255). The concept of subtlety has a central place in the eighteenth century hermeneutic tradition. It is a concept with several dimensions. It refers to a certain disposition: a delicacy of mind. It also refers to a certain attitude: a sensitivity to the unique authenticity of others. And, finally, it refers to a certain quality of professional skills: meticulousness and precision. Hans-Georg Gadamer, the great philosopher of German hermeneutics, has explained how in the hermeneutics tradition of Pietism three forms of subtlety were distinguished. The first is the *subtilitas intelligendi* which is related to the activity of creating and understanding a certain image. The *subtilitas explicandi* refers to the quality of being able to explain to one's self and to others what has been understood. Finally, a *subtilitas applicandi* is a prerequisite for the right implementation of the understood in real life. Gadamer has strongly emphasized that distinguishing these aspects should not lead to separate them from each other. Understanding takes place in explaining, understanding and explaining take place in practical application (Gadamer, 1990, p. 212).

Considering care and support as interpretative practices, we may come to understand the value of subtlety, a virtue which is closely connected to the skills of hermeneutical competence that should be practiced in an attitude of imagination and anticipation. The interweaving of this virtue, those skills and this attitude is the central characteristic of the practice of an inclusive anthropology in care for persons with intellectual disabilities.

REFERENCES

Bleidick, Ulrich, 'Die Behinderung im Menschenbild und hinderliche Menschenbilder in der Erziehung von Behinderten.' In *Zeitschrift für Heilpädagogik* 41 (1990) 8, p. 514-534.

Bleidick, Ulrich, Hagemeister, Ursula, *Einführung in die Behindertenpädagogik. Band I, Allgemeine Theorie der Behindertenpädagogik*. Stuttgart/Berlin/Köln (Kohlhammer) 1992[4].

Clegg, Jennifer, 'Beyond Ethical Individualism.' In *Journal of Intellectual Disability Research* 44 (2000) 1, p. 1-11.

Edwards, Steven D., 'The Moral Status of Intellectually Disabled Individuals.' In *The Journal of Medicine and Philosophy* 22 (1997) p. 29-42.

Gadamer, Hans-Georg, *Gesammelte Werke, Bd. 1, Hermeneutik I: Wahrheit und Methode. Grundzüge eine Philosophischen Hermeneutik*. Tübingen (J.C.B. Mohr) 1990[6].

Gennep, A. van, 'Visies op verstandelijke handicap en op de zorg voor mensen met een verstandelijke handicap.' In: G.H. van Gemert, R.B. Minderaa (red.), *Zorg voor verstandelijk gehandicapten*. Assen (Van Gorcum) 1993, p. 3-21.

Hall, Douglas John, *Imaging God. Dominion as Stewardship*. Grand Rapids (Wm.B. Eerdmans Publishing Co.) 1986.

Horne, Brian L., 'Person as Confession: Augustine of Hippo.' In: Christoph Schwöbel, Colin E. Gunton (Eds.), *Persons, Divine and Human*. Edinburg (T&T Clark) 1991, p. 65-73.

Jantzen, Wolfgang, "Praktische Ethik" als Verlust der Utopiefähigkeit-Anthropologische und naturphilosophische Argumente gegen Peter Singer.' In: *Behindertenpädagogik* 30 (1991) 1, p. 11-25.

MacMurray, John, *Persons in Relation*. London (Faber and Faber Ltd.) 1961.

Mataheru, Mattijn, *Vroegtijdige onderkenning van gedragsstoornissen bij verstandelijk gehandicapten. Een ontwerp voor een protocol om het risico van hardnekkige problemen in de omgang met verstandelijk gehandicapten te taxeren*. Amersfoort (Vereniging's Heeren Loo) 1995.

Meininger, Herman P., 'Respect: weg naar wederkerigheid.' In: *Vlaams Tijdschrift voor Orthopedagogiek* 15 (1996) 4, p. 18-30.

Meininger, Herman P., ' . . . als uzelf.' *Een theologisch-ethische studie van zorg voor verstandelijk gehandicapten*. Amersfoort (Vereniging's Heeren Loo) 1998.

Moltmann, Jürgen, *Gott in der Schöpfung. Ökologische Schöpfungslehre*, Gütersloh (Chr. Kaiser) 1993[4].

Moltmann, Jürgen, *In der Geschichte des dreieinigen Gottes. Beiträge zur trinitarischen Theologie*, München (Chr. Kaiser) 1991.

Moltmann, Jürgen, *Trinität und Reich Gottes. Zur Gotteslehre*. München (Chr. Kaiser) 1980.

Reinders, J.S., 'Wat niets kan worden, stelt niets voor.' Mensen met een ernstige verstandelijke handicap in het licht van de hedendaagse gezondheidsethiek. Een kritische uiteenzetting. Amersfoort ('s Heeren Loo) 1996.

Schönberger, Franz, 'Sind Geistigbehinderte amoralische Wesen? Randbemerkungen zur abendländischen Vernunftethik.' In: Jürg Blickenstorfer, e.a., *Ethik in der Sonderpädagogik*. Berling (Marhold) 1988, p. 279-299.

Schwöbel, Christoph, 'God's Goodness and Human Morality.' In: *Nederlands Theologisch Tijdschrift* 43 (1909)2, p. 122-138.

Siegenthaler, Hermann, *Anthropologische Grundlagen zur Erziehung Geistigschwerstbehinderter*, Bern/Stuttgart (Paul Haupt) 1983.

Siegenthaler, Hermann, *Menschenbild und Heilpädagogik. Beiträge zur Heilpäda gogischen Anthropologie*, Luzern (Edition SZH) 1993.

Taylor, Charles, *The Ethics of Authenticity*. Cambridge/London (Harvard University Press) 1991.

Zizioulas, J.D. 'On Being a Person. Towards an Ontology of Personhood.' In Chr. Schwöbel, C.E. Gunton (eds.), *Persons, Divine and Human*, Edinburgh (T&T Clark) 1991, p. 33-46.

Zizioulas, J.D., 'Communion and Otherness.' In *Sobornost: The Journal of the Fellowship of S. Alban and S. Sergius* 16 (1994) 1, p. 7-19.

Zizioulas, J.D., 'Human Capacity and Human Incapacity: A Theological Exploration of Personhood.' In *Scottish Journal of Theology* 28 (1975) p. 401-448.

Zizioulas, J.D., *Being as Communion. Studies in Personhood and the Church*. New York (St. Wladimir Press) 1975.

Defining and Assessing Spirituality and Spiritual Supports: A Rationale for Inclusion in Theory and Practice

William C. Gaventa, Jr., MDiv

SUMMARY. The 1992 definition of mental retardation by the AAMR (American Association on Mental Retardation) was the first termination and classification system in developmental disabilities to include the importance of spiritual supports. This paper proposes that "spirituality" be further developed to become the fifth dimension of assessment process. It explores definitions of spirituality, four rationales for enhanced inclusion of spirituality in assessment and supports, and several implications,

William C. Gaventa, Jr. is Coordinator, Community and Congregational Supports, and Assistant Professor Co-Terminous, Elizabeth M. Boggs Center on Developmental Disabilities of the Robert Wood Johnson Medical School, University of Medicine and Dentistry of New Jersey. Bill is a certified supervisor in Clinical Pastoral Education and serves in volunteer roles as Executive Secretary of the Religion and Spirituality Division of the AAMR and Co-Editor of the *Journal of Religion, Disability, & Health*.

Many of the ideas in this presentation and paper were first developed in a chapter entitled "Defining and Assessing Spirituality and Spiritual Supports: Moving from Benediction to Invocation" that is being published in an AAMR book edited by Greenspan, S., and Switsky, H.J. (in press) *What Is Mental Retardation?: Ideas for an Evolving Disability Definition.* Washington, DC: American Association on Mental Retardation. It is an interdisciplinary reflection on the revised 1992 Termination and Classification System, and possibilities for its future use and evolution.

[Haworth co-indexing entry note]: "Defining and Assessing Spirituality and Spiritual Supports: A Rationale for Inclusion in Theory and Practice." Gaventa, William C. Jr. Co-published simultaneously in *Journal of Religion, Disability & Health* (The Haworth Pastoral Press, an imprint of The Haworth Press, Inc.) Vol. 5, No. 2/3, 2001, pp. 29-48; and: *Spirituality and Intellectual Disability: International Perspectives on the Effect of Culture and Religion on Healing Body, Mind, and Soul* (eds: William C. Gaventa, Jr. and David L. Coulter) The Haworth Pastoral Press, an imprint of The Haworth Press, Inc., 2001, pp. 29-48. Single or multiple copies of this article are available for a fee from The Haworth Document Delivery Service [1-800-342-9678, 9:00 a.m. - 5:00 p.m. (EST). E-mail address: getinfo@haworthpressinc.com].

and some of the challenges which spirituality brings to understandings of professional ethics, identity, and practice. *[Article copies available for a fee from The Haworth Document Delivery Service: 1-800-342-9678. E-mail address: <getinfo@haworthpressinc.com> Website: <http://www.HaworthPress.com> © 2001 by The Haworth Press, Inc. All rights reserved.]*

KEYWORDS. Spirituality, mental retardation, intellectual disability, assessment, supports, meaning, coping, self-determination, cultural diversity

DEFINING AND ASSESSING SPIRITUALITY AND SPIRITUAL SUPPORTS: A RATIONALE FOR INCLUSION IN THEORY AND PRACTICE

This strand of sessions exploring Spirituality and Disability at the conference of the International Association for the Scientific Study of Intellectual Disability is a first in the history of the IASSID. The theme of the conference is "From Theory to Practice." My purpose in this presentation and paper is to provide a rationale for a serious, intentional exploration of the role of spirituality in both theory and practice in services and supports for people with intellectual disabilities and their families. There are a number of challenges in that task. One is to build a bridge and partnership between "science" and "religion" or "faith." A second is building a framework that recognizes my own American roots, but speaks to an international audience. The third is also to recognize and speak from my Judeo Christian background in a way that is clear about my history and experience, but also may relate to perspectives based within other major traditions of faith, religion, and spirituality. So let me start with a reference point that should be familiar to many within this international association, i.e., the revised definition of mental retardation published by the American Association on Mental Retardation in 1992.

A BEGINNING WITH PROMISE

From the perspective of those involved in ministries and spiritual supports with people with mental retardation and their families, the 1992 AAMR revised definition of mental retardation was a major step forward in the recognition of the holistic, multidimensional nature of the lives of persons with mental retardation and human life in general. It has been a controversial definition, because of its movement away from easily standardized tests. But for many, it was a more accurate and truthful expression of the wondrous complexity of individuals, relationships, and environments, for at least four reasons:

1. It affirms a more holistic view of people with mental retardation, confirming the experience of many researchers, practitioners, and families that strengths in some areas of a person's life may exist side by side with limitations in others. Hence, many who have witnessed, affirmed, and experienced people primarily in terms of their gifts and strengths, along with their significant limitations in other areas, can see in that definition an affirmation of the value of each person.
2. It recognizes the importance of opportunity and experience for learning and development. Hence, those who have seen people with developmental disabilities change, learn, and grow through participation in faith communities have a way of defining the importance of opportunity and practice. It also then opens the door to talk about what it might mean to be "at risk" in a spiritual sense, e.g., never having opportunities to experience love, to be part of a community of faith, or connected with sources of hope?
3. It correctly states that limitations and function must be explored in the context of culture, because different cultures and settings place different values and interpretations on what might appear to be the "same" human ability, disability, or behavior.
4. By including the importance of spiritual awareness and supports in a discussion of the implications of using supports, and delineating a distinction between spiritual awareness and intelligence (Chapter 9), the definition took a major step towards creating a context for dialogue and collaboration between people, organizations, and communities who provide supports from different theoretical foundations or starting points, especially that of spirituality.

Having started from the "scientific" side represented by the 1992 definition let me re-start this discussion from the other end of this bridge. A "spiritual" or "theological" definition might first start with the fundamental affirmation that all human beings have within them a spark of divinity, or, as in the Judeo-Christian perspective, are created in the image of God. An attempt to assess, understand, or define a person with intellectual disabilities and functional limitations from a spiritual or theological dimension immediately puts one in touch with fundamental questions of meaning and purpose. (Gaventa, 1997) What does it mean to be human? What and who is "God," that which is sacred or divine, in this person's life (and my own?) Why is there difference? Why is there pain or suffering? What is the purpose of that person's life and my own in relation to them? And how are we connected to each other in our understanding of humankind?

The 1992 definition answers those fundamental questions in a decidedly Western and certainly American context through the affirmed values of independence, productivity, and integration. From a spiritual perspective, those values, respectively, are "answers" to the universal questions of identity (Who am I?), purpose (Why am I?), and community (Whose am I?). From that perspective, the recognition of spiritual awareness as a dimension of human life and the importance of spiritual supports was an important first step, but just that . . . a first step. In the years since 1992, there has been a growing body of literature and research articulating the importance of spirituality and the nature of spiritual supports in a wide variety of human services. Rather than being one of four "implications" of the concept of supports, I submit that the definition needs to be broadened to reflect spirituality as a basic dimension of human life. That's what this presentation will now turn its attention toward doing. To use a distinction from the world of faith and the varieties of prayer, this presentation will advocate for moving the role of spirituality from an important "benediction" onto the 1992 definition to the more active role of being regularly "invoked" as a part of assessments, care, and supports.

REVISING THE DEFINITION:
THE FIFTH DIMENSION

Put simply, the basic way in which the definition needs to be revised is not to change the definition per se, but to add "spirituality" as the fifth dimension in its multi-dimensional approach diagnosis, classification, and supports:

Current:

Dimension I: Intellectual Functioning and Adaptive Skills
Dimension II: Psychological/Emotional Considerations

Dimension III: Physical Health and Etiology Considerations
Dimension IV: Environmental Considerations

Proposed:

Dimension V: Spiritual Considerations

Researchers, theorists, and practitioners define spirituality in a huge variety of ways. The most helpful definition in my opinion comes from another interdisciplinary, multi-dimensional approach to diagnosis and supports which views spirituality as one of seven dimensions of assessment and care. (Fitchett, 1993) Fitchett defines the "spiritual" as "the dimension of life that reflects the need to find meaning in existence and in which we respond to the sacred." Working with nurses and other health care professionals in the late 1980's in Chicago, they developed what was envisioned as a "functional approach" to spiritual assessment, an approach that focused more on how a person makes meaning in his or her life than on what that specific meaning is.

As defined by multiple researchers (Carder, 1984; Fitchett, 1993; Larson, 1994) spirituality is also seen as a broader category than religion. There is a spiritual dimension to life that may or may not be experienced or lived out in the context of a specific faith community. Adherence to, or membership in, a particular faith community might be what one would call a "substantive" approach to spirituality, i.e., specific beliefs with a defined community of practice. The implication for both research and practice is that assessment needs to be more sophisticated than simply whether or not one goes to church, synagogue, or temple, wants to go or not, and has the appropriate supports to do so.

In Fitchett's 7 x7 Model for Spiritual Assessment, spirituality is one of seven dimensions of assessment that need to be explored in a holistic process (see Table 1).

In the Spiritual Dimension, there are seven areas or tools to be used to assess a person's spiritual life: (1) Belief and meaning, i.e., major beliefs, sense of purpose, symbols, affiliation; (2) Vocation and obligations, e.g., a sense of calling, duty; (3) Experience and emotion, i.e., experiences of the sacred, divine, or demonic, and feelings or interpretations associated with those experiences; (4) Courage and growth, or how is a person open to change in beliefs based on experience?; (5) Ritual and practice, i.e., what are the rituals and practices associated with

TABLE 1

HOLISTIC ASSESSMENT	SPIRITUAL ASSESSMENT
Biological (Medical) Dimension	Belief and Meaning
Psychological Dimension	Vocation and Obligations
Family Systems Dimension	Experience and Emotion
Psycho-Social Dimension	Courage and Growth
Ethnic/Racial/Cultural Dimension	Ritual and Practice
Social Issues Dimension	Community
Spiritual Dimension	Authority and Guidance

the beliefs and meaning systems of this person; (6) Community, e.g., is the person a part of a formal or informal community of shared belief, meaning, ritual, or practice? What is the style of participation?; and (7) Authority and guidance, or, where does the person find authority for the beliefs and practices. Where does a person look for guidance when needed? Does that authority come from within or without? (Fitchett, 1993).

The reason for outlining the comprehensiveness of this particular model is to articulate a rationale for including the spiritual as one of the five dimensions in the AAMR system rather than subsuming it under one of the other four. Spirituality is, for many, related to *intellectual functioning and adaptive skills*, but one of the basic issues in the recognition of the spiritual needs and gifts of person with mental retardation is that spirituality is too often equated with doctrine or intellectual understanding (AAMR, 1992). Spirituality can also be expressed in all of the adaptive skills in the current definition. For other theorists, spirituality would seem to be emotional or psychological, yet in the current definition, this dimension is more closely related to identification of mental health issues. Other researchers (Larson, 1994) have done a comprehensive exploration of the historical way that spirituality or religiousness was too often dismissed as a "symptom" of mental illness without recognizing the ways it is also a powerful contributor to mental and emotional health. There is increasing research that illuminates the impact of spirituality on *physical health*, from the perspectives of prevention, wellness, and recovery as well as support for coping with chronic conditions. (Wallis, 1996, Matthews, Larson, and Barry, 1993). Fourth, as part of the dimension of *"Environmental Considerations,"* spirituality is clearly related to culture, community, and inclusion. The Fitchett model is much more sophisticated than the AAMR Assessment process in exploring the multiple dimensions of family, environment, and social contexts.

Thus, I would argue that spirituality does not "fit" under one of the current dimensions, but rather is a "pervasive" dimension that needs to be assessed in dynamic relationships with the other four. To frame the argument more positively, there are at least four reasons for including and expanding the role of spirituality as a dimension of the assessment and diagnostic system:

First, it recognizes that the spiritual is a dimension of human experience in which people grow and develop as in other areas of life (Westerhoff, 1976; Fowler, 1981; Webb-Mitchell, 1993). Where does one find love, meaning, and hope, or experience mystery, trust, awe, the sacred or divine . . . or the opposites of those?

Second, as Fitchett and others have outlined, spirituality is a major way of finding meaning, coping, understanding, changing, and motivating. Whether or not one believes that spirituality is "substantive" or "real" part of human experience, we cannot ignore its functional role.

Third, spirituality is a major component of cultures and communities. If we are to be "culturally competent" as professionals, we have to recognize and utilize the spiritual beliefs of individuals, communities, and cultures as part of the context in which people live their own lives. If we want to mobilize inclusive, natural supports and empower "consumers" and communities, understanding and collaboration with sources of spiritual supports is crucial (Heifitz, 1987; Gaventa, 1997; Dudley, 1993; Landau-Stanton, 1993).

Fourth, spirituality is a dimension of life and experience which begs for the honoring of "consumer" choice and empowerment (Hoeksema, 1995). Indeed, in the theoretical base of self-determination, "spirituality" is articulated in its four value framework of "freedom, authority, support, and responsibility" as a "responsibility," i.e., an assumption that spirituality is a primary way of utilizing one's gifts in service to the wider community. (Nerney and Shumway, 1996)

Let's explore some of the research and theoretical foundations for each of these four reasons for more comprehensive inclusion of spirituality in assessment and practice.

EXPANDING THE RATIONALE FOR A DIMENSION OF SPIRITUALITY

"Expanding a rationale for spirituality" may sound to some like a contradiction in terms, but the four areas are only a brief summation of the theoretical research and practice that is taking place in a number of disciplines and areas of human service in relation to the importance of spirituality as a dimension of holistic assessment and comprehensive supports.

Spirituality as a Dimension of Life and Growth

The seminal work on spiritual and faith development was begun by Westerhoff (1976) and Fowler (1981), whose work was based on developmental theories of Erickson. Wolfensberger (1979, 1982) pointed to fundamental theological, spiritual, and prophetic themes in services and supports with people with mental retardation. Providers and researchers began to hear about the work of Jean Vanier and the L'Arche communities, the intentional (and international) communities of care and support which are based on a spiritual understanding of human growth in community. People from many faith, spiritual, and theoretical backgrounds have known the capacity of persons with mental retardation to appreciate and exhibit a spiritual life, but the systems of definition and classification made that very difficult to affirm in research and theory. One only has to remember the graphic passage in *The Man Who Mistook His Wife for A Hat* (Sacks, 1987, pp. 178-186) in which Oliver Sacks defines the difference between the Rebecca he saw in the examination room and the same person he saw outside in a garden, communing with the world of nature in a way in which the assessment instruments could not explain. Coles (1990) explored the spiritual lives of children, followed by Webb-Mitchell in an explicit examination of children with disabilities (1993).

In *The Right to Grow Up* (Summers, J. (Ed.), 1986, I worked on an interdisciplinary model that utilized Westerhoff's understanding of faith development to explore the dimensions of spiritual and religious growth. In his model, spirituality (or faith) comes as "styles":

1. Experienced faith . . . in which individuals experience communities and times of love, trust, joy, and celebration;
2. Affiliative faith, characterized often by emotional attachment to a set of beliefs and a particular community of faith, where the authority resides in the community;
3. Searching, a style or period in one's spiritual journey characterized by questioning, searching, and experimentation in beliefs, communities of faith, and social action; and

4. "Owned" faith, a coming to one's own faith style, often character-ized by a renewed sense of the importance of spiritual practice and the importance of shared community.

Others have taken the more explicit and elaborate stages of faith as defined by Fowler and applied them to their work and experience with persons with different levels of mental retardation (Schurter, 1994). In a more recent work, Schurter utilizes levels of support needs to delineate ways to provide support functions with individuals with mental retarda-tion dealing with grief, death, and dying (Schurter, 1998). Glenda Prins, a chaplain in Rochester, utilized a theoretical model for spiritual diag-nosis developed by Lex Tartaglia (Landau-Stanton and Clements, 1993) in development of a spiritual life plan for each person served by her agency. The Tartaglia framework is particularly thought provoking for the ways it combines both experience of fundamental spiritual ques-tions and interpretation of that experience (see Table 2).

Prins (1994) utilized this framework to assess spiritual strengths and needs, and plan ways to increase experiences of safety, hope and trust-fulness, enhance a sense of belonging, acceptance and community, en-courage experiences of self worth, and strengthen a sense of personal value, purpose, or meaning. The plan utilized religious activities as ex-pressions of those dimensions as appropriate to each individual, but it is evident that the model does not necessarily have to include religious participation, ritual, or belief.

Spirituality as Meaning, Purpose, and Coping

Besides the model and research of Fitchett cited earlier, there are lit-erally hundreds of spiritual assessment instruments and research mod-els that have been developed to take into account the ways in which people utilize spirituality and religious faith to describe purpose and meaning in their lives. Some encourage spiritual growth as a means of motivation and coping. Others articulate the impact of spirituality and religion on illness prevention and recovery, i.e., healing, or understand-ings of healing that do not involve cure or recovery. (Matthews, Larson, Barry, 1993, Larson and Larson, 1994; Fairer, 1995; Smith, 1998) There has been extensive research on the importance of spirituality in the areas of aging, hospice care, HIV-AIDS, children, addictions, and mental illness. Those studies have led in many service systems, such as the US Joint Commission for the Accreditation of Health Organiza-tions, to standards of care that ask how spiritual needs of patients are

TABLE 2

Spiritual Diagnosis	Image of God	Experience	Existential Question	Experience	Image of God	Spiritual Diagnosis
Fear	Unpredictable Capricious Chaotic	Mistrust Victimization Helplessness Passivity	"Am I safe?" "Is my world a threat or opportunity?"	Hope, Courage, Active agency Opportunity	Trustworthy Reliable	Faith
Alienation	Vengeful Divisive	Social stigma External judgement, Rejection Estrangement	"Do I belong?"	Social acceptance, Communion, Embracement	Loving, Inclusive	Community
Guilt	Punishing Judgmental	Internalized stigma Personal responsibility for illness	"Am I worthy?"	Grace Repentance	Merciful, Compassionate	Reconciliation
Despair	Withholding Silent Absent	Meaninglessness Death anxiety Non-being	"Am I valued?" "Do I leave a legacy?" "Did my life make a difference?" "Am I content?" "Regretful?"	Vocation Purpose Creativity Meaning	Blessing Affirming Revealing	Providence

met in hospitals and hospices. They have also led to headline-making national conferences on the relationships between spirituality and healing in medicine, and to large numbers of alternative therapies with spiritual components in addition to increased attention to more traditional spiritual practices. There has been some recent theoretical and research attention on spirituality in developmental disabilities, but most of it has focused on spirituality and religion as a framework for coping and meaning by families (e.g., Haworth, Hill, Glidden, 1996). The careful delineations of experience and interpretation in both Fitchett and Tartaglia point the way to a variety of ways that research and practice could address spiritual gifts and needs of persons with intellectual disabilities and other developmental disabilities.

Spirituality and Culture

With the growing imperative of public policy to be "culturally competent" in the design and delivery of services and supports, the role of spirituality, particularly as described in the 7 × 7 Model by Fitchett, becomes abundantly clear. What are the belief systems of this individual, family, and community? What meaning is placed on "disability" or even "diagnosis?" Can the community see and develop a place for this individual to live out their own sense of vocation, or, as we say, to make a contribution. What are the rituals and practice, the holidays and traditions, that give meaning to people's lives, particularly in periods of transition or change (Hornstein, 1997). How do people grow and change? How might attitudes and practices be changed, particularly ones that may be traditional but neglectful or harmful? Where are the experiences of community, belonging, and affirmation? Who does one turn to for guidance?

For many service providers and researchers, the question is even more fundamental: What authority figures might we turn to in a given community to gain the trust needed in order to develop accurate assessments and effective supports? Whether one frames the research and planning in terms of eco-cultural issues (Gallimore, Weisner et al., 1989), community associations (McKnight and Kretzmann, 1993), family issues in particular cultures (Rogers-Dulan, 1998), religious identity (Moran and Weiner, 1991), or concerns for the "optimum environment that provides opportunities, fosters well-being, and promotes stability" (AAMR, 1992), the issue of effective and ethical practice begs for respect of the spiritual traditions and centers of cultural life and for enhanced research that can lead to more effective collaboration and practice. That importance is amplified when practitioners suspect or hear experiences of the ways in which spirituality or religion can be used to hurt and harm as well as to help. One can dismiss spirituality as "bad" or "hurtful" but a deeper understanding may provide advocates, providers, and friends with alternative interpretations and/or practices within that same spiritual tradition.

Spirituality as Choice and Self-Determination

A number of researchers and practitioners have pointed to the importance of congregations and spiritual communities as pathways and supports into community life and relationships (Amado, 1993). One of the more common dilemmas faced by consumers, advocates, and supporters is that spiritual and religious rights may be affirmed in policy, but not supported in practice. In the United States, the fear of "proselytizing" and of violating the "wall between church and state" point to real issues that need careful exploration, but they are not the same as recognizing, affirming, and supporting the importance of spirituality as a dimension of life for people with (or without) mental retardation. (Gaventa, 1993)

In an article that originated in his role as consultant and mediator to resolve a lawsuit about proselytizing and agency policy, Hoeksema

(1995) outlined the importance of respecting and supporting religious freedom in the group home context. He pointed the way towards responsible guidelines for policies and practices in those settings, and, as such, helped focus the question of spirituality away from professional belief and practice to respecting citizenship and choice.

In the years since, the importance of assisting individuals to make choices, and the relationship between choice, control, self-determination and well-being has received increasing attention in professional literature and practice. The theoretical basis for the growing self determination movement, i.e., the values of freedom, authority, support, and responsibility, demonstrate the importance of values at the heart of professional practice. Values are closely related to spirituality, as defined by the meaning and purpose that is interpreted from experience. When it comes to spiritual expression, it does not take much imagination to recognize the ways in which spirituality becomes a field of potential choices waiting to be supported. Freedom to choose one's needed supports (Do I want to go to church today?), authority and power to make choice real (It's your job to help me get there, as we have defined it in your job description, whether or not it is your faith tradition. And it is more important to me that you be here on Saturday morning to go to synagogue than it is to help me go through yet another diagnostic and assessment process.), and support (maybe it does not have to be a paid job to support my decision, but my paid staff can help me develop connections and friendships at the local *(you fill in the blank)*, which is my major spiritual community). A paper at the 1998 AAMR National Conference (Gleason, 1998) pointed to the importance placed on spiritual supports by one agency which became convinced that this was a major way to actively enhance the quality of life for the people they served.

One of the intriguing components of spirituality in these theoretical underpinnings of self-determination is that it is connected to the fourth value of "responsibility," i.e.,:

> the acceptance of a valued role in a person's community through competitive employment, organizational affiliations, spiritual development and general caring for others in the community, as well as accountability of spending public dollars in ways that are life-enhancing for persons with disabilities. . . . The intense over-regulation of programs and the setting of goals and objectives to meet the needs of the human service system more than the aspirations of people with disabilities, have conspired to prevent people with disabilities from truly contributing to the associational

life of their communities, the spiritual life of our churches and synagogues, and the cultural and artistic life of our cities and towns. (Nerney and Shumway, 1996)

These four theoretical foundations for expanding "spirituality" to a dimension of assessment and practice point to two other reasons that focus more on professional practice than to an assessment of another individual or the development of a plan for needed supports. These are ethics and professional identity.

The crucial role of ethics in research, assessment, practice, and supports is evident in the fact that there is within the IASSID an active Special Interest Research Group on ethics. The assumptions one makes about human life and growth, the ways we all discern and manufacture meaning and values, the influence of our cultural traditions on fundamental perceptions of what is right and wrong, and our political affirmations about what it means to be citizen as well as consumer of services all shape the way we approach ethical questions in our work, issues with specific individuals in specific situations, and systemic issues of policy and resource allocation. The spiritual assumptions, foundations, and imperatives for ethical decision-making and practice cannot be ignored.

The second reason is professional honesty, identity, and development. It may be hard to talk about, but if we are honest, it is the spiritual gifts, struggles, and pains of people with disabilities and their families that have "called" many of us into vocations which have provided meaning and purpose for professional caregivers. The questions, which "they," i.e., our clients or consumers, face about independence, productivity, and integration, are also our own journeys into meaning, values, and motivation. One could make a strong case for seeing people with disabilities as "our" spiritual guides. Seeing the diversity of spiritual gifts in different cultural contexts enriches our own. Being "professional," whether diagnostician, provider, planner, or policy maker, is a position of incredible power that we are struggling to share with those who say they are now community member and citizen, not just consumer and client. The challenge to professional identity and power, in an age of empowerment, is one that is much broader than health and human services. In a book which comes from international work being done in participatory research and planning in economic development, Robert Chambers systematically outlines the challenge to professionals in its very title: *Whose Reality Counts? Putting the first last.* (Chambers, 1999) In many ways, we are being pushed toward a much older definition of "profess-ional," one who is at least clear and open about values, loyalties, and willingness to share what one has to help fulfill a vision of community (Gaventa, 1993, 1998).

FROM RATIONALE TO IMPLICATIONS: THE CHALLENGE OF RECOGNIZING SPIRITUALITY AS A DIMENSION OF ASSESSMENT AND SUPPORTS

There are number of ways in which the expansion of the dimension of spirituality could impact other areas of the 1992 AAMR Definition and Classification System. Some which quickly come to mind are things such as assessing and defining gifts and strengths more carefully, exploring understandings of vocation, calling, and responsibility to the wider community, and providing clearer guidelines and models for assessing spirituality, supporting choice, and changing practice.

The parallels between discussions of the difficulty of assessing spirituality (substantive experiences or beliefs vs. functional, interpretations of meaning and experience) and the difficulty of assessing mental retardation or intellectual disability may or may not be obvious. Is mental retardation or intellectual disability a substantial characteristic of some people's experience, i.e., real unto itself, or is it interpretation? Is it substance, experience, or interpretation, and what is the function of the definition at all levels? To whom is a definition real, by whom are its implications experienced, and how is it interpreted?

In the Judeo-Christian tradition, the power of "naming" is a gift given to Adam and Eve as a way of continuing the process of creation through ordering and naming that which God had created. (Note that in almost every one of the first six days, God paused to decide whether or not the newly named part of creation was "good.") There is also the fascinating account in the "second" story of creation in Genesis 2 that the naming of all the animals, birds, and fish was part of the process of bring order but also of finding a helper as his partner, for "it is not good that man should be alone." But there were also boundaries . . . some things shall not be touched or named. The tree of life was one. And later, it was God, who refused to give an answer to Moses' question and search for a clear classification, by stating "I am Who I am."

That is one way of saying that a spiritual perspective on the process of defining and classification may need to recognize there are some parts of life which defy naming, dominion, and control, and which instead, beg for respect and honor. Matters of the spiritual have been difficult to "classify." That may be a function of their "observable, measurable, material" elusiveness, and/or it may be a function of our innate awareness of their power, which we sometimes call "irrational." Wherever one stands, there remains the Biblical question of whether and how the naming does more than bring dominion and control. It also asks where is the helpful partner, and whether or not we can respect depths of experience that call for wonder and mystery. We need to ask how the process of naming and classification functions? Whom does it help? How?

But the second question for the definition and classification system comes from the Latin root of the word "assessment," which meant to "sit next to." (Hilsman, 1997). If we do indeed need to "sit next to" in order to see and understand what is real in and for another, to be with them in their context, to listen to self report, observe behavior and skills, and then assess and plan, that raises even further the question of the power of definition and the power of the definer. "Who owns the definition?" is a question that is much more fundamental than whether it is AAMR's, APA's, CEC's, or, "IASSID's." If, through defining, you own or have power over the person, then whose is the responsibility? If we sit next to, in order to observe and assess, are we honest about the impact of the event on the observer as well as the observed?

A number of years ago, when we still used the categories of mild, moderate, severe and profound retardation, I literally played around with the implications of this question in a devotional meditation by exploring the levels of feeling in the observer that might correspond to those levels of disability. We, the observer, can respond to difference in both positive and negative ways. My proposed schemata looked like this (see Table 3).

Again, please understand, I was not, nor do I propose, that this is an "objective" reality. But a serious exploration of spirituality in assessment and practice calls for an honest assessment of what happens to both parties, "client" as well as "professional."

As we evolve toward another paradigm that affirms the crucial importance of community embeddedness (which can be supported or hindered by professional practice, but not provided), and a paradigm of "empowerment," then the importance of the ethical questions of naming and definition are even further heightened. Is a definition or classification, then, one that is functional and useful, for the individual, his or her particular community, and for his or her potential community?

TABLE 3

Level of Disability	Positive Response in Observer	Negative Response in Observer
Mild	Curiosity	Anxiety
Moderate	Amazement	Fear
Severe	Wonder	Terror
Profound	Mystery	Despair

A VIEW TOWARD THE FUTURE

My temptation was to call this section a "prophetic" look at the future, but a self-named prophet is, by definition, not one. The argument in this presentation for more comprehensive recognition, inclusion, and use of the spiritual dimension of human life in a system of diagnosis, classification, and supports is based on the personal experience of many I know, on sound theory from a wide variety of theoretical perspectives, and, increasingly, on a significant body of research. Whether one recognizes and affirms the spiritual dimension as a substantial (i.e., real?) dimension of human experience, a functional process of discerning meaning and purpose in human experience (which is also real), a recognition of the role of spirituality in culture and community, or as a consumer right and choice that needs to be respected and honored, the theoretical foundation is there.

That recognition raises some interesting questions. How might we talk about "adaptive spirituality." What does or might it mean to be "spiritually competent"? Or, even more provocatively, what does it mean to be "spiritually retarded" or "spiritually disabled?" Those questions raise the specter of the spiritual abuse very quickly, but if one goes back to the Tartaglia model, we all know in personal experience or professional practice what it means to be "disabled spiritually." To be caught in despair, to have lost hope, to have little experience of love or affirmation, to lack trust in anyone: we have seen that in others or been there personally, and the potential "client population" is much broader than that defined by "mental retardation." Many people I know will give witness to the incredible spiritual strengths of people we label "retarded" in other dimensions of their life.

The real prophets in our time are the self-advocates who raise the question outlined in the previous section: Who owns the definition and defining process? What is the function? How is it helpful, and to whom? Most self advocates in the United States say it is time to change the definition and the name that is used here. To most, it feels hurtful. If "naming" is about the development of understanding and mastery over chaos, but also about the creation of a helpful partnership, it is time to hear and recognize the call for a new kind of partnership between "consumer" and "clinician" that is based on citizenship if not on congregation.

That partnership would not just be between "consumer" and "clinician," but also between American perspectives and the rest of the world, where the emerging paradigm is either "mental disability" or "intellectual disability." It would put limitations in intellectual functioning, paired with other life skill limitations, more firmly within the paradigm of "intellectual, physical, emotional, and, perhaps, spiritual disabilities."

Whatever the decisions about the construct and diagnostic process, the future will continue to see more research and practice focused on the integration of the spiritual dimension in human services and caregiving. Congregations and faith communities in America continue to grow as a major source of community inclusion and natural supports, guided advocates and friends. They are also increasingly compelled and called to do so by families and self-advocates who are asking for the same opportunity to give voice and practice to their spiritual identity and journey.

The challenge to clinical and professional practice is then multi-dimensional as well. There is first the question of developing effective models and processes for assessing the spiritual dimension as part of any diagnostic and support planning process. The models are there from other areas of human service, which are, in many instances, much farther ahead. Given the current focus of research in a number of health care disciplines and areas of need on the role of spirituality and faith, one hope is that same kind of research could develop in the area of developmental disabilities in relation to what the AAMR Classification System calls primary, secondary, and tertiary prevention, and, more proactively, on the quality of lives of individuals and families.

Second, there is the question of how professional caregivers then help provide appropriate spiritual supports. Is it just a job for the "religious professional?" The nursing profession has long ago decided that paying attention to spiritual care was one of the components of their responsibility (Schoenbeck, 1994). Research, training, and writing is being done in many disciplines other than theology and pastoral care about the responsibilities of professionals to pay attention to the spiritual dimension of the lives of the people they serve. Those include social work (Dudley and Helfgott, 1990), occupational therapy (Farrar, 1995); psychology (Heifitz, 1987), and psychiatry and medicine (Larson, 1994). The barriers cited to more effective practice include concern about "church/state" separation, understandings of "professional" identity, lack of knowledge, lack of funding, and personal history (Dudley, 1990; Hoeksema, 1995; Heifitz, 1987). All of those have and can be addressed if we believe this to be a crucial dimension of care (Gaventa, 1993). But more work needs to be done on what it means to be a "spiritual clinician" (Hilsman, 1997) or, borrowing a term from supported employment, a "church coach" (Gaventa, 1996).

The final challenge then comes back to professional identity as well as practice. Does "profess-ional" mean the one in control of a body of knowledge, the fixer, and the expert or does it mean one who possesses some knowledge but also "professes" a commitment to walk alongside others as well as "sit next to them" in an assessment process, and a belief in the capacity of the partnership to sustain and perhaps even overcome the challenges which are faced together. Professionals from many fields, both "scientific" and "religious," have been much better at naming, diagnosing, and classifying that they have been at fixing or healing, and especially at sustaining or supporting.

So let me conclude with the same hope and thesis with which this paper began: the importance of expanding the systems of definition, classification, and supports to include systematic assessment of the spiritual dimensions of the people we serve, with both the belief and knowledge that this can contribute to more holistic understandings of individuals, families, and communities, and more effective, and collaborative, systems of support and care. Spirituality is a dimension of life to be invoked, explored, and tapped as well as one that can give a blessing, or benediction, to a service and support plan that assumes, sometimes, it is already complete.

REFERENCES

Carder, M. (1984) Spiritual and religious needs of mentally retarded persons. *The Journal of Pastoral Care.* XXXVIII (2).

Chambers, R. (1999) *Whose reality counts? Putting the first last.* London: Intermediate Technology Publications.

Coles, R. (1990) *The spiritual life of children.* Boston: Houghton Mifflin.

Coulter. D. (1994). Spiritual supports in the 1992 AAMR system. *NAPMR Quarterly.* Fall/Winter.

Dudley, J. & Helfgott, C. (1990). Exploring a place for spirituality in the social work curriculum. *Journal of Social Work Education.* 26, pp. 287-294.

Dudley, J. & Millison, M. (1992). Providing spiritual support: A job for all hospice professionals. *The Hospice Journal.* 8(4). pp. 49-66.

Dudley, J., Smith, C., & Millison, M. (1995). Unfinished business: assessing the spiritual needs of hospice clients. *The American Journal of Hospice and Palliative Care.* March/April, 1995. pp. 30-37.

Farrar, J. (1995) *Client's spirituality and religious life: Challenging the scope of occupational therapy practice.* Unpublished Thesis. Tufts University.

Fitchett, G. (1993). *Spiritual assessment in pastoral care: a guide to selected resources.* Decatur: Journal of Pastoral Care Publications, Inc.

Fitchett, G. (1993). *Assessing spiritual needs: A guide for caregivers.* Minneapolis: Augsburg/Fortress Press.

Fitchett, G. (1996). The 7x7 model for spiritual assessment. *Vision.* (Newsletter of National Association of Catholic Chaplains). March. pp. 10-11.

Fowler, J. (1981) *Stages of faith. The psychology of human development and the quest for meaning.* San Francisco: Harper and Row.

Gallimore, R., Weisner, T., Kaufman, S., Bernheimer, L. (1989) The social construction of ecocultural niches: Family accommodation of developmentally disabled children. *American Journal on Mental Retardation.* 94 (3), 216-230.

Gaventa, W. (1986) Religious ministries and services with adults with developmental disabilities. In Summers, J. (Ed.) *The right to grow up: An introduction to adults with developmental disabilities.* Baltimore: Brookes.

Gaventa, W. (1993). Gift and call: recovering the spiritual foundations of friendships. In A. Amado (Ed.) *Friendships and community connections between people with and without developmental disabilities.*(pp. 41-66). Baltimore: Brookes.

Gaventa, W. (1993) From belief to belonging to belief: Trends in religious ministries and services with people with mental retardation. *Disability Rag/Resource.* September/October. pp. 27-29.

Gaventa, W. (1996) Honoring diversity through spirit and faith. *Impact.* 9 (3). University of Minnesota, pp. 10-11.

Gaventa, W. (1997) "Pastoral care with people with disabilities and their families: An adaptable module for introductory courses." In *Thematic conversations regarding disability within the framework of courses of worship, scripture, and pastoral care.* Dayton: National Council of Churches Committee on Disabilities.

Gaventa, W. (in press) Recovering the meaning of professional. *Frontline Initiative.*

Haworth, A., Hill, A., Glidden, L. (1996) Measuring the religiousness of parents of children with developmental disabilities. *Mental Retardation.* 34 (5), 271-279.

Heifitz, L. (1987) Integrating religious and secular perspectives in the design and delivery of disability Services. *American Journal of Mental Retardation.* 25, 127-131.

Hilsman,G. (1997) Spiritual pathways: One response to the current standards challenge. *Vision.* June, 1997. 8-9.

Hoeksema, T. (1995) Supporting the free exercise of religion in the group home context. *Mental Retardation.* 33(5), 289-294.

Hornstein, B. (1997) How the religious community can support the transition to adulthood: A parent's perspective. *Mental Retardation.* (35) 6. 485-487.

Kretzmann, J. & McKnight, J. (1993) *Building communities from the inside out: A path toward finding and mobilizing a community's assets.* Evanston: Northwestern University.

Larson, D. and Larson, S. (1991) Religious commitment and health: Valuing the relationship. *Second Opinion*. July. 27-40.

Larson, D. & Larson, S. (1994) *The forgotten factor in physical and mental health: What does the research show?* Rockville: National Institute of Healthcare Research.

Laundau-Stanton.J, Clements,C., Tartaglia, A., Nudd, J. & Espaillat-Pina,E. (1993) Spiritual, cultural, and community systems. In Landau-Stanton, J. & Clements, C. (Eds.) *AIDS: Health and mental health. A primary sourcebook*. (pp. 267-298) New York. Bruner/Mazel.

Matthews,D., Larson, D., & Barry,C. (1993) *The faith factor: An annotated bibliography of clinical research on spiritual subjects*. Rockville: National Institute for Healthcare Research.

Moran, M. & Weiner,K. (1991) *Spiritual and faith community integration needs of catholic developmentally disabled adults*. Holyoke, MA: Bureau for Exceptional Children, Inc.

Nerney, T. & Shumway, D. (1996) *Beyond managed care: Self determination for people with disabilities*. Concord, NH: University of New Hampshire.

Prins, G. (1994) Spiritual Life Plan. Boston: AAMR National Conference.

Rice, D & Dudley, J. (1997). Preparing students for the spiritual issues of their clients through a self-awareness exercise. *The Journal of Baccalaureate Social Work*, 3(1), pp. 85-95.

Rogers-Dulan, J. (1998) Religious connectedness among urban African American families who have a child with disabilities. *Mental Retardation*. (36)2, 91-103.

Sacks, O. *The man who mistook his wife for a hat and other clinical tales*. New York: Harper and Row, 1987.

Schoenbeck, S. (1994) Called to care: addressing the spiritual needs of patients. *The Journal of Practical Nursing*. September. 19-23.

Schurter, D. (1994) Guidance for the journey–Fowler's stages of faith as a guide for ministry with people with mental retardation. In *A mutual ministry: Theological reflections and resources on ministry with people with mental retardation and other disabilities*. Denton, TX: Denton State School. 35-43.

Schurter, D. (1998) A developmental model for grief in people with mental retardation. San Diego: AAMR National Conference.

Smith, J. *Parents' perceptions of the spiritual needs of their adult child with mental retardation*. Forthcoming Dissertation. Lewis University.

Sommer, D. (1994) Exploring the spirituality of children in the midst of illness and suffering. *The ACCH Advocate*. 1(2). pp.7-12.

Wallis, C. (1996). Faith and healing. *Time Magazine*. June 24, 1996. pp. 58-64.

Webb-Mitchell, B. (1993) *God plays the piano too: The spiritual lives of disabled children*. New York: Crossroad.

Westerhoff, J. (1976) *Will our children have faith?* New York: Seabury Press.

Wolfensberger, W. (1979) An attempt toward a theology of social integration of devalued/handicapped people. Information Service, 8 (1), Publication of Religion Division, AAMR, 12-26.

Wolfensberger, W. (1982) An attempt to gain a better understanding from a Christian perspective of what "mental retardation" is. *National Apostolate with Mentally Retarded Persons Quarterly*. 13 (3) 2-7.

II. SPIRITUALITY AND INTELLECTUAL DISABILITY AROUND THE WORLD: CULTURAL AND RELIGIOUS PERSPECTIVES ON HEALING MIND, BODY, AND SOUL

Judaism and the Person with Intellectual Disability

Joav Merrick, MD, DMSc
Yehuda Gabbay
Hefziba Lifshitz, PhD

SUMMARY. The cornerstones of Judaism are the people (Am Israel), the land (Erez Israel) and the Written and Oral teachings (Torah Israel). Judaism is not only a religion, but a way of life. Not only for special events, like circumcision, bar mitzvah, weddings or funerals, but every

Joav Merrick is Medical Director, Division for Mental Retardation, Ministry of Labour and Social Affairs, P.O. Box 1260, IL-91012 Jerusalem, Israel (E-mail: jmerrick@aquanet.co.il). Yehuda Gabbay is a Talmudic student at the Netivot Chaim Yeshiva, Kiryat Malachi, Israel. Hefziba Lifshitz is Lecturer at the School of Education, Bar Ilan University, IL-52900 Ramat Gan, Israel.

[Haworth co-indexing entry note]: "Judaism and the Person with Intellectual Disability." Merrick, Joav, Yehuda Gabbay, and Hefziba Lifshitz. Co-published simultaneously in *Journal of Religion, Disability & Health* (The Haworth Pastoral Press, an imprint of The Haworth Press, Inc.) Vol. 5, No. 2/3, 2001, pp. 49-63; and: *Spirituality and Intellectual Disability: International Perspectives on the Effect of Culture and Religion on Healing Body, Mind, and Soul* (eds: William C. Gaventa, Jr. and David L. Coulter) The Haworth Pastoral Press, an imprint of The Haworth Press, Inc., 2001, pp. 49-63. Single or multiple copies of this article are available for a fee from The Haworth Document Delivery Service [1-800-342-9678, 9:00 a.m. - 5:00 p.m. (EST). E-mail address: getinfo@haworthpressinc.com].

49

minute of the life of a Jewish person. Judaism is not just an aspect of a Jew's life, but the totality of it. Torah operates all the time, covers every aspect of life and is unchangeable, unamendable and absolute. Torah is so deep spiritually that a lifetime is not enough to understand it fully. Rambam, a great scholar, said: "For one who gladdens the heart of these unfortunate is similar to the Divine, "as it says," To revive the spirit of the lowly and to revive the heart of the contrite." Jewish Law and scholars over time have stressed the need for education, acceptance and obligations towards persons with intellectual disability. This presentation will discuss the Jewish aspects of intellectual disability. *[Article copies available for a fee from The Haworth Document Delivery Service: 1-800-342-9678. E-mail address: <getinfo@haworthpressinc.com> Website: <http://www.HaworthPress.com> © 2001 by The Haworth Press, Inc. All rights reserved.]*

KEYWORDS. Intellectual disability, Jewish Law, Halacha, Israel

Judaism is based upon a set of beliefs, which has become the possession of all mankind. The Jewish faith does not claim that the Jews were the first to worship one God. Our tradition is based on what we call the law of the sons of Noah, the law that is the foundation of an universal ethical religion:

- The worship of God
- The ban on murder
- The ban on theft
- The ban on incest and sex aberrations
- The ban of eating "the limb of the living" or cruelty to animals
- The ban on blasphemy
- Justice–the establishment of courts, judges and a system of equity

Judaism received the ten commandments from God at Mount Sinai and they guide the Jews in his everyday life:

- I am Hashem, your God, who delivered you from the land of Egypt, from the house of slavery
- You shall not recognize the gods of others before My presence. You shall not make yourself a carved image nor any likeness of that which is in the heavens above, or of that which is on the earth below, or of that which is in the water beneath the earth. You shall

not prostrate yourself to them nor shall you worship them; for I am Hashem, your God–a jealous God, remembering the sins of fathers upon children, to the third and fourth generations of my enemies, but showing kindness for thousands of generations to those who love Me and who keep my commandments
- You shall not take the Name of Hashem, your God, in vain oath; for Hashem will not absolve anyone who takes him name in a vain oath
- Remember the Sabbath day to sanctify it. Six days you are to work and accomplish all your tasks. But the seventh day is Sabbath to Hashem, your God; you may not do any work–you, your son, your daughter, your manservant, your maidservant, your animal, and the convert within your gates–for in six days Hashem made the heavens, the earth, the sea and all that is in them, and he rested on the seventh day. Therefore, Hashem blessed the Sabbath day and sanctified it
- Honor your father and mother so that your days may be lengthened upon the land which Hashem, your God, gives you
- You shall not kill
- You shall not commit adultery
- You shall not steal
- You shall not bear false witness against your neighbor
- You shall not covet your neighbor's house. You shall not covet your neighbor's wife, nor his manservant, nor his maidservant, nor his bull, nor his donkey, nor anything that is your neighbor's.

Historically, Judaism never separated belief from performance, so in the Torah (the written law or Bible and the oral law or Talmud) the commandment to believe in God is not stated differently from the laws on Kashrut or lending money, but over the years other religions and ideas began to influence a number of Jews and one of our great rabbis, Rambam (Rabbi Moses Maimonides (1135-1204), formulated the Thirteen Principles of Faith, which have received universal acceptance among the Jewish people:

1. Belief in the existence of God
2. Belief in God's unity
3. Belief in God's incorporeality
4. Belief in God's eternity
5. Belief that God alone is to be worshipped
6. Belief in prophecy
7. Belief in Moses as the greatest of the prophets

8. Belief that the Torah was given by God to Moses
9. Belief that the Torah is immutable
10. Belief that God knows the thoughts and deeds of men
11. Belief that God rewards and punishes
12. Belief in the advent of the Messiah
13. Belief in the resurrection of the dead.

Before turning to the main point of this presentation it warrants to explain the meaning of the Bible or Torah of Israel. The Torah is not only a number of history books, but a guide explaining how we should live and conduct our lives. One of the great rabbis once wrote to one of his students about the Torah of Israel:

> The Torah for us is the existence and breath of the Jewish nation. Like air for breathing, without it no living thing can exist on earth, so too the Torah for a believing and non-believing Jew. He has no right to spiritual existence for even one hour without it, because it is the core of our spiritual lives and the Torah is the loving altar upon which millions of Jews poured their blood and gave their souls as their mouths were full of their life-song in their declaration of "Hear O Israel, the Lord is our God, the Lord is one."

The Torah gives the Jew vision and purpose in life, a feeling of supremacy and special purpose in life for the superior mission he must accomplish and with the superior strength of Torah he overcomes failures during his lifetime. From this it can be seen that the Torah instead of a history book is more of a guidebook for life from which the Jew can draw his power.

THE ESSENCE OF JUDAISM

Judaism is a religion based on the performance of commandments. The are 613 commandments, mitzvot or religious obligations of which 248 (corresponding to the number of members in the human body) are positive commandments of things one must do and 365 (corresponding to the number of days in the year) prohibitions.

These mitzvot (most are related to farming, the temple and criminal law) cannot all be kept today and even a rabbi in the third century called Simlai (Steinberg, 1975) tried to reduce the Jewish faith to its essence this way:

- 613 commandments were imparted to Moses
- Then came David and reduced them to eleven, even as it is written (Psalms XV):
- "Lord, who shall sojourn in Thy tabernacle?
- Who shall dwell on Thy holy mountain?
- He that walketh uprightly and worketh righteousness,
- And speaketh truth in his heart:
- That hath no slander upon his tongue,
- Nor doeth evil to his fellow
- Nor taketh up a reproach against his neighbor:
- In whose eyes a vile person is despised,
- But he honoreth them that fear the Lord;
- He that sweareth to his own hurt and breaketh not his word;
- He that putteth not out his money on interest,
- Nor taketh a bribe against the innocent.
- He that doeth these things shall never be moved."
- Then came Isaiah and reduced them to six, even as it is written (Isiah XXXIII:15):
- "He that walketh righteously, and speaketh uprightly;
- He that despiseth the gain of oppressions,
- That shaketh clear his hands from laying hold on bribes,
- That stoppeth his ears from hearing of blood
- And shutteth his eyes from looking upon evil."
- Then came Micah and reduced them to three, even as it is written (Micah VI:8):
- "It hath been told thee, O man, what is good,
- And what the Lord doth require of thee:
- Only to do justly, and to love mercy, and to walk humbly with thy God."
- Then came Isaiah once more and reduced them to two, as it is said (Isiah LVI:1):
- "Thus saith the Lord;
- Keep ye justice, and do righteousness."
- Then came Amos and reduced them to one, as it is said (Amos V:4):
- "Seek ye Me, and live."

Another great Sage of Judaism, Rabbi Hillel, who lived in the second century BCE, put it very plainly to a convert, who asked to be taught all the Torah, while standing on one foot. Hillel told him: "Love your neighbor as yourself. All the rest is commentary. Go now and learn."

Every Jewish boy, from his birth to the age of thirteen years, is called a minor or baby, but after his Bar Mitzvah at 13 years he is known as an adult or man. At this age he begins to be responsible for his own actions and obliged to perform and fulfill mitzvot. For a Jewish girl the age of reason begins at the age of 12 years.

Now we come to the question of how Jewish Law, also called Halacha, regards the person, who already has passed the age of thirteen, but with an intellectual disability. When studying the Torah, both the Bible or five books of Moses and the Talmud (completed during the fifth century CE), you will not find a definition of mental retardation, developmental disability or intellectual disability.

On the other hand the Talmud mentions other disabilities, such as derangement, deafness and blindness.

THE JEWISH VIEW OF DEAFNESS

In Jewish law deaf people were in the same category as minors and the insane or imbecile, meaning that they could not be held responsible for their actions. The Rabbis considered deaf people to be more like children than like the insane. On the other hand, the Rabbis realized that the deaf person was mentally superior to the imbecile.

In the Talmud (Sabbath 153a) there is a discussion on whom to leave your purse with if Sabbath fall, while traveling on the road. In this passage the Rabbis grade in decending order the minor, the deaf-mute and the imbecile.

The deaf person was excluded from public life and could not serve as a witness, lead public prayer or be involved in property transactions, but on the other hand it was accepted that the deaf person could be married and divorced using sign language, if both parties understood. Marriage could be to both a normal person or another deaf-mute person. The details of the manner in which a marriage or a divorce should take place was laid down in great detail and has been the subject of a special responsa (Encyclopaedia Judaica, 1972).

In the past century the stigma of mental retardation has been removed from the deaf persons. In Vienna there was a school for teaching deaf children to speak and read Hebrew and the principals tried already in 1864 to get the acceptance of the deaf persons in the Jewish community (Strassfeld & Strassfeld, 1976), but they talked to "deaf ears." In 1963 the Rabbinical Court of London, Beth Din, ruled that deaf persons can be called to the Torah reading and recite the blessings (Strassfeld & Strassfeld, 1976).

THE JEWISH VIEW OF BLINDNESS

The blind person in The Jewish law is regarded as fully normal and most of the legal and religious restrictions placed upon him are due to the physical disability. The Bible twice warns us not to mistreat the blind, once with the statement "You shall not insult the deaf or place a stumbling block before the blind" (Leviticus 19:14) and next with "Cursed be he who misdirects a blind person on his way" (Deuteronomy 27:18).

On the other hand there are also some ambivalence in the Bible, because Itzak, our forefather, being visually impaired in old age was easely deceived by his wife and son. A blind Cohen or priest is disqualified from Temple service: "No man of your offspring throughout the ages who has a defect shall be qualified to offer the food of his God . . . no man who is blind, or lame, or has a limb too short or too long . . . he shall not profane these places sacred to Me" (Leviticus 21:17-23).

The blind person can be called to the Torah and recite the blessings, he can testify as a witness and even though is was not recommended, it was also not forbidden for a totally blind person to act as a Judge.

DEFINITION AND LEGAL ASPECTS
OF INTELLECTUAL DISABILITY

In Erez Israel during the Hadrianic persecutions Jews were killed, sold as slaves or deported or fled to mainly Babylon and organized Jewish life was on the verge of extinction. The process was halted in 138, when Hadrian died and his successor, Antoninus Pius, took over. A new academic Sanhedrin was established in Galil under the predicency of Rabbi Simeon ben Gamliel, whom Antoninus Pius regarded as the supreme head of the Jews.

Schools and religious life was revived and reached its peak under the guidence of Rabbi Simeon ben Gamliel's son, Judah, called the Rabbi or teacher (135-217). He realized that "the calm could not last forever" and therefore set out to create an instrument to preserve Jewish Law and tradition for generations to come. This is the Mishnah, devided in six orders and each order devided into a total of 63 tractates, which again is divided into chapters and paragraphs covering all aspects of Jewish life. In the following centuries the scholars of Judaism studied and investigated the Mishnah and this work with their commentaries is called the Gemara (or completion). The Mishnah (completed around the year 200) and the Gemara (completed around the year 500) together makes up the Talmud (or to study), which has a Babylonean and Jerusalem version. This Talmud is studied every day by Jews around the world.

The Talmud puts the person with intellectual disability into a category together with the deaf and the minor, as in the Mishnah (Talmud, Hagigah 3b) on who is bound to appear at the Temple:

> Mishnah. All are bound to appear (at the Temple), except a deaf man, an imbecile and a minor, a person of unknown sex, a hermaphridite, women, unfreed slaves, the lame, the blind, the sick, the aged and one who is unable to go up on foot. Who is a minor? Whoever is unable to ride on his father's shoulders and go up from Jerusalem to the Temple Mount. This is the view of Beit Shammai.
>
> But Beit Hillel say: "Whoever is unable to hold his father's hand and go up from Jerusalem to the Temple Mount, for it is said: Three regalim."

In the following discussion of the Gemara each word is discussed and the definition of the imbecile has the following explanation (Talmud, Hagigah, 3b), which can be seen as a rather functional description:

> Our Rabbis taught: Who is (deemed) an imbecile? He that goes out alone at night and he that spends the night in a cemetery, and he that tears his garments. It was taught: R. Huna said: They must all be (done) together. R. Yohanan said: Even if (he does only) one of them. What is the case? If he does them in an insane manner, even one is also (proof). If he does not do them in an insane manner, even all of them (prove) nothing? Actually (it is a case where) he does them in an insane manner. But if he spent the night in a cemetery, I might say: He did (it) in order that the spirit of impurity might rest upon him. If he went out alone at night, I might say: He was seized with lycanthropy. If he tore his garment, I might say: he was lost in thought, But as soon as he does them all, he becomes like (an ox), who gored an ox, an ass and a camel, and becomes (thereby) a muad (forewarned gorer) in regard to all (animals). R. Papa said: If R. Huna had heard of that which is taught: Who is (deemed) an imbecile? One that destroys all that is given to him; he would have retracted, would he have retracted only with regard to the (case of the) man who tore his garment, because it resembles this (case) or would he have tetracted with regard to all of them ? It remains undecided.

The Rambam, Rabbi Moses Maimonides, one of the great leaders of Judaism and a physician, wrote many books commenting on the Torah, on philosophy, Jewish Law, science and especially medical books. His books are still studied in many universities today and by many Jews every day. He was one of the first scholars, who specially refered to and described the person with intellectual disability (he referred to them as *petti* or in plural *pettaim*, meaning *feebleminded*). He looked upon persons with intellectual disability as people and even if they are not complete in their body or mind, their position should not suffer.

He ruled in his work (Rambam) that the testimony of a petti or shoteh could not be accepted in the Court:

> . . . one must testify about what has already happened and there is concern that what the witness might, at that moment, imagine is really true, actually is not and was exchanged for something else and he will not testify about what he saw at first.

So the Bible, in spite of the differences, really emphasize that the person with intellectual disability is really like any person despite his deficiencies.

The Rabbis have also determined that even though a person with intellectual disability is exempt from mitzvot or commandments it is absolutely forbidden to use him for the violation of any commandment.

OBLIGATION TO EDUCATE THE PERSON WITH INTELLECTUAL DISABILITY

The definition of intellectual disability in different writings and various types indicates the question of educational obligations and commandments. In the case of severe intellectual disability, where it is clear the person is not intelligent and there is no chance of progress in intelligence the person is exempt from commandments and entitled to full societal protection. But there is a difference of opinion regarding mild intellectual disability.

A parent is required to teach his children the Torah and to see that they receive formal instruction in Jewish religious studies. This is a fulfillment of the command from the Bible: "And you shall teach them (these words of the Torah) to your children . . . " (Deut. 11:19). The Talmud also obligates the father to teach his son a skill, because he who does not teaches the child to steal.

The Talmud has the following advice concerning students that cannot grasp what they learn (Talmud, Taanith 8a):

> Resh Lakish said: If you see a student to whom his studies are as hard as iron, it is because he has failed to systematize his studies, as it is said, and one do not whet the egde. What is his remedy? Let him attend the school even more regularly, as it is said, then must he put to more strength; but wisdom is profitable to direct. (The latter words indicate) how much more profitable would his efforts be if he had originally systematized his studies. Thus for example, Resh Lakish made it his practice to repeat in systematic order his studies forty times corresponding to the forty days during which the Torah was given and only then would he come before R. Yohanan. R. Abba ben Abbahu made it his practice to repeat in systematic order his studies twenty-four times corresponding to the (twenty-four books which embody) the Torah, the Prophets and the Hagiographa and only then would he come before Raba.

The Gemarah continues and says that if you see a student whose studies are difficult for him like iron that is a sign that no one is explaining to him face to face. We see here another example of the relationship, where the teacher influences the student's absorption of the material.

The commandment of Bible study and educating children is for its own sake and not for preparing for matriculation or the intellectual ability of the child. This is a commandment for its own sake and it is the obligation of the father. Therefore, in any case it is the father's duty to educate him and teach him even if there is no chance the child will live and even if we know with clarity that he will live for only one year there is still the obligation for the father to educate him, because the Bible does not stipulate what type of child should be taught.

Now that we know there is an obligation for the father to educate, we need to find out if the community has a responsibilty to educate a child with intellectual disability. The Gemara gives us the answer through the decree of Rabbi Yehoshua Ben Gamla (Talmud, Baba Bathra 21a):

> . . . for but for him the Torah would have been forgotten from Israel. For at first if a child had a father, his father taught him, and if he had no father he did not learn at all. By that (verse in the Scripture) did they guide themselves? By the verse, "And ye shall teach them to your children." Laying emphasis on the word "ye." They then made an ordinance that teachers of children should be ap-

pointed in Jerusalem. By that verse did they guide themselves? By the verse, "For from Zion shall the Torah go forth." Even so, however, if a child had a father, the father would take him up to Jerusalem and have him taught there, and if not, he would not go up to learn there. They therefore ordained that teachers should be appointed in each prefecture and that boys should enter school at the age of sixteen or seventeen. (They did so) and if the teacher punished them they used to rebel and leave the school. At length Yehushua ben Gamla came and ordained that teachers of young children should be appointed in each district and each town and that children should enter school at the age of six or seven.

Rab said to R. Samuel ben Shilath: Before the age of six do not accept pupils; from that age you can accept them and stuff them with Torah like an ox. Rab also said to R. Samuel ben Shilath: When you punish a pupil, only hit him with a shoe latchet. The attentive one will read (of himself) and if one is inattentive, put him next to a diligent one.

We see from the above that it is the duty of the community and not limited to the father-son relationship to teach our children. Therefore each child has the right to an education and it is not dependent upon his intellectual level.

And in our time, we were instructed by one of the most eminent teachers, Rabbi Moshe Feinstein, that it is the duty of the father to assist, through the community, the local authority or govenment to establish institutions for special education in order to teach children with intellectual disability.

METHOD FOR THE DIAGNOSIS
OF INTELLECTUAL DISABILITY

Rambam described the method of "check him three times alternately if he says to them not not not and yes yes yes . . . " The questions that should be asked are "testing him about fruit that are in season only in the summer, and asking him in the winter time if he wants for them to pick him fruit of that kind or not." These questions, a recipe for understanding the absurd, were developed, such as if he wants to wear a summer outfit in the winter and the opposite, and if he wants to divorce his mother and other statements of this kind.

Additional ways to check intelligence and consideration of those suspected of intellectual disability are through tasks like "collecting and throwing away a walnut and it's leftovers." If we were to give a child a real walnut and a rock that appeared to be a walnut, and the child threw away the rock and kept the walnut then we would assume he has understanding, knowledge, memory, awareness and the ability to determine and act out. Or we could send him to shop for something from the marketplace in order to see if he knows how to negotiate and if he is involved with reality.

These tests checked not only the given situation, but also the thought process of the child. To find out if he does what is being told him, if he knows how to care for things, if he has shame and if he has presence of mind. Even through faith can a child's intellect be checked. If asked if he knows to whom he is blessing and he points to the heavens then he understands there is a base for faith and there is a creator, who gave the commandments and we are fulfilling his commandments.

METHOD FOR TEACHING THE CHILD
WITH INTELLECTUAL DISABILITY

It is written in the Shulchan Aruch (a book of Jewish Law): "Even a baby who does not know how to read you cannot throw him out of there, but must allow him to sit with the others because he might understand." Together with this, the Talmud informs us of the connections and the difficulties of intelligence socially and educationally in the higher grades and it gives an example: One thousand students enter for Bible study, one hundred of them go on to Mishnah, which is more difficult, ten of them go on to Gemara, a very high and difficult level, one of them goes on to become a teacher, which is the highest level.

A classic example of teaching children with intellectual disability is given in the Talmud (Talmus, Eruvin 54b):

R. Preida had a student to whom he would have to repeat each lesson four hundred times before he understood it. One day (R. Preida) was required to leave and attend to a certain matter involving a mitzvah. Before leaving. He taught (the student) the usual four hundred times, but he still did not grasp the lesson. (R. Preida) asked him, "Why is today different?" (The student) answered him, "From the very moment they told master that there is a mitzvah matter for him to attend, my attention was diverted, because every moment I said that now the master will get up and leave: now the master will get up and leave." (R. Preida) said to him, "Pay attention and I will teach you." He taught him again (another) four hundred times. A Heavenly voice emanated and asked (R. Preida), "Do you prefer that four hundred year be added to your life, or that you and your generation merit the life of the World to come?" (R. Preida) replied: "That I and my generation merit the life of the World to come." The Holy One, blessed is He, said to them: "give him both this and this."

Rabbi Preida showed that dedication and individual attention are the necessary ingredients for a teacher to succeed with his students.

The Jewish tradition does not accept the ban of students from studying the Torah and looks upon such behaviour as if someone stealing from his friend. Rabbi Yehuda said anyone preventing Torah from a student is as if he stole from the inheritance of our forefathers. Rabbi Shmuel Eliezer Halevy warns teachers and rabbis, who say a student has no reasoning and is not worthy of Bible study, or that it is impossible to teach him, that they are stealing the inheritance of our forefathers. Here again we see the concern and the importance of education regardless irrespective of the student's educational or intellectual level.

The Rabbis also as a part of the learning method determined the size of the special class. Primary school-age children should have twenty-five students to a class, but for students with learning disabilities the class should not have more than eight students (for comparison, the average size of a special education class for learning disabled in Israel today is twelve students per class, mild intellectual disabiilty, eight-ten students per class; severe intellectual disability, six-eight students per class and autistic children five students per class).

Throughout the history of the Jewish people the communities all over the world found special approaches for learning disabled students. As an example in Altuna, where the community decided that those children who appear to not have the ability to study Gemara should have hired students to teach them. Also from the community of Mudina (in the year 1597) it was reported that industrious students and those who excelled were assisting the weaker ones.

MARRIAGE AND DIVORCE AND THE PERSON WITH INTELLECTUAL DISABILITY

Regarding marriage, the criterion for validity is the minimal understanding level (called daat kpeutot or the level of a six year normal child) and comprehension of the specific act. If the person with intellectual disability has a level of that kind and understands the significance of marrying, then the marriage ceremony is valid.

However, Jewish Law or Halacha also recognizes situations in which a person functions at a level lower than "daat kpeutot," but is nevertheless capable of understanding the significance of the act of marriage. This possibility was described by Rabbi Raphael Lipman Halperin, (the "Oneg YomTov," Poland,19th century) and cited by Farbstein (11):

> ... a man with a speech defect making his words extremely difficult to understand, and even people used to his company do not always understand his speech, and his mind is very weak, and does not even know how to count, he does not understand the meaning of divorce at all, and it never occurred to him to divorce, because never, since his birth, has he known that divorce exists in the world, and he does not even know anything about the Torah. And whatever he does, he does only because he has habitually seen others doing these things . . . (Halperin)

> This man's acts of marriage are valid acts, because we have seen that he can adopt acts that he regularly sees in his environment; this person has the legal status of one who is intelligent, because when something is explained, it makes sense to him. (Farbstein)

In other words, the Rabbis take into account situations where people with intellectual disability may exhibit greater and lesser abilities in different areas of functioning being very deficient in one domain, while in another being able to understand complex actions. Therefore Rabbi Halperin maintained, that if the person understood the meaning of being married, even if the person did not understand the ceremonial act of marriage, the act itself will be considered valid. This position has become Halacha.

In Jewish law divorce is more complex than marriage. To wed, "it is enough that he understands that he is taking a wife, and it is not necessary for him to understand that the Act of Marriage is performed by means of something with monetary value (the marriage contract) (Farbstein, 1995). Divorce, on the other hand, entails mutual consent and the husband's initiating of the Bill of Divorcement or Get. The husband must understand not only that he is divorcing his wife, but also that it is the Get, which puts into effect the divorce. If he understands both points, the divorce is valid; if he does not, the divorce has no legal standing. Like the man, the woman has to understand the significance of the Get, which means that she has to leave her husband and make no efforts to reside with him again.

CONCLUSION

It seems that Judaism and Jewish Law have had a functional approach to intellectual disability and a flexible view on the complex issues involved during a long history. Education and respect for the person with ID also seems to have been important points of interest.

To illustrate the respect Rabbis gave to the person with intellectual disability, the story of Hazon Ish (Avraham Yeshayahu Karelitz, 1878-1953) comes to mind: As the teacher, scholar and author of many books he received many visitors and one day a father came to visit him together with his son with intellectual disability. The father entered the study of Hazon Ish and when his son entered the Hazon Ish stood up and gave respect to the other visitor. The father did not understand why the great Rabbi had stood up and wondered if another visitor had entered the room without his notice. When the father asked the Hazon Ish why he had stood up, Hazon Ish answered that he had risen out of respect for his son.

REFERENCES

The Babylonian Talmud. Seder Moed, Sabbath 153a.
The Babylonian Talmud. Seder Moed, Hagigah 2a.
The Babylonian Talmud. Seder Moed, Hagigah 3b.
The Babylonian Talmud. Seder Moed, Taanith, 8a.
The Babylonian Talmud, Seder Moed, Eruvin, 54b.
The Babylonian Talmud, Seder Nezikin, Baba Bathra, 21a.
Encyclopaedia Judaica.(1972) Jerusalem: Keter, 5:1419-20.
Farbstein M. (1995). Legal principal and clarification of the daat concept and laws concerning the soteh. Jerusalem: Shaar Hamispat Institute, (Hebrew).
Rambam. Mishneh Totah, Laws of Evidence, 69:9-10.
Steinberg, M. (1975) Basic Judaism. New York: Harvest Book, 13-4.
Strassfeld S, Strassfeld M, eds.(1976) The second Jewish catalog. Philadelphia: The Jewish Publication Society of America, 151-66.

Islam and the Person
with Intellectual Disability

Mohammed Morad, MD
Yusuf Nasri, MD
Joav Merrick, MD, DMSc

SUMMARY. Islam, as a religion, makes a distinction between the person with intellectual disability and mental disorder, but both are found legally incompetent in the Koran and the Hadith. The society according to Islam is obliged to assess, assist and respect the person with intellectual disability and give the person an equal life chance. Mohammad, the Prophet, implied the importance of child welfare, education, well-being, and supporting children other than your own, all which can be seen as the expression of Islamic compassion. Islam recognizes the right of the needing person for help and assistance, as God tells us in the Qur'an (Koran): "And in their wealth there is acknowledged right for the needy and the destitute" (51:19). In Islamic tradition, it has been stated that the best therapy is the one directed to enhance the health of the person, his psyche and spirit, in order for him to fight illness. His environment should be beautiful, filled with music and people he likes. This presentation will

Mohammed Morad is Family Physician, Department of Family Medicine, Ben Gurion University, Beer Sheva, Israel. Yusuf Nasri is Family Physician, Department of Family Medicine, Ben Gurion University, Beer Sheva, Israel. Joav Merrick is Medical Director, Division for Mental Retardation in Israel, Ministry of Labour and Social Affairs, Jerusalem, Israel (E-mail: jmerrick@aquanet.co.il).

Address correspondence to: Mohammed Morad, MD, Department of Family Medicine, Ben Gurion University in Beer Sheva, Andarta 7/12, Ramot Beer-Sheva, Israel MD (E-mail: morad-62@barak-online.net).

[Haworth co-indexing entry note]: "Islam and the Person with Intellectual Disability." Morad, Mohammed, Yusuf Nasri, and Joav Merrick. Co-published simultaneously in *Journal of Religion, Disability & Health* (The Haworth Pastoral Press, an imprint of The Haworth Press, Inc.) Vol. 5, No. 2/3, 2001, pp. 65-71; and: *Spirituality and Intellectual Disability: International Perspectives on the Effect of Culture and Religion on Healing Body, Mind, and Soul* (eds: William C. Gaventa, Jr. and David L. Coulter) The Haworth Pastoral Press, an imprint of The Haworth Press, Inc., 2001, pp. 65-71. Single or multiple copies of this article are available for a fee from The Haworth Document Delivery Service [1-800-342-9678, 9:00 a.m. - 5:00 p.m. (EST). E-mail address: getinfo@haworthpressinc.com].

65

describe the Islamic tradition and how it deals with and looks upon persons with intellectual disability. *[Article copies available for a fee from The Haworth Document Delivery Service: 1-800-342-9678. E-mail address: <getinfo@haworthpressinc.com> Website: <http://www.HaworthPress.com> © 2001 by The Haworth Press, Inc. All rights reserved.]*

KEYWORDS. Intellectual disability, Islam, history

The Prophet Mohammad (571-632) was born in Mecca. In 610, he declared the Islam. He died in 632, after changing the whole tribal society of the Arabic Pennisula, and preparing it for bringing the light to people of the medieval period (from the 7th-13th centuries) in all aspects of life (Anwar, 1973).

From the beginning, the Islam paid great attention to medical care and medicine as a discipline. The Prophet Mohammad himself established the first military field hospital for injured soldiers during his first battles in the 5th century.

By practicing Islamic laws, the Moslem should be able to attain spiritual health and wealth, say the Moslem scientists (Muchtar, 1995). The Koran (Qur'an) and the Hadith (the science of Islamic tradition, applying particularly to the Sunna, the actions, sayings, virtues, opinions and ways of life of Mohammad), emphasize the recently documented evidence of the benefit of spiritual practices in improving all aspects of health. In Surah Moon, "God deprecates those who are careless in their prayers and offer them only for show," and the blessed Prophet said, "Prayers are certainly health promoting." In another citation, "O, mankind! There hath come to you a direction from your Lord and healing for the (diseases) in your hearts and for those who believe, a Guidance and a Mercy" (Surah Yunus, verse 57). In Surah Bani Israil it is even clearer: "We send down in the Qur'an that is a healing and a mercy to those who believe." The Prophet said (Hadith): "We did not send down any disease, unless we have sent down the remedy with it."

And in the Qur'an a verse tells us "Everything good that happens to you is from God, everything bad that happens to you is from your own actions." The awareness of God increases in illness and man come closer to God, while realizing his own weakness.

ISLAMIC SOURCES AND INTELLECTUAL DISABILITY

The Qur'an and the Hadith (Anwar, 1973) constitute the origins and codices of the Islamic believers' behavior in different spheres of existence; spiritual-religious, and social, including: intra-family and inter-family relationships, the individual norms of persons toward each other and toward God. Reward and punishment in life and after death are the main legislative executive steps provided by God. The four sources: The Holy Qur'an; the Hadith (The Prophet's sayings), Al-Ijmah and Al-qias, that constitute the science of Islamic religion (Al-fiqh) (Anwar, 1973), provide the way for the Moslem to enter heaven. The view of Islam on the well-being of man indicates he is to abstain from forbidden things and to do everything he is commanded by God to do.

Islam is engaged in the care of man even before he is born (Mahmoud, 1990, Human rights in Islam, 1999). The fetus is considered a human being and his legal rights are incoporated in the Islamic law very deeply. The parents have to care for the health of their children in order to bring to this world healthy children and the role of the physician is to find solutions to protect the mother and her child from suffering before the soul is put in the fetal body. As it is said: "Nor take life, which God has made sacred except for a just cause." (The Qur'an, Surah Bani Israil 17:33)

Avoidance of consanguineous marriages is recommended in the Qur'an and the Hadith. The Prophet (Hadith) said that healthy family life and understanding of parents are obligatory for the health, physically and mentally, of the child. After birth, the child is in the care of his mother unless it harms his health and interests. The parents are obliged to be patient with their children and teach them, because learning is a duty of the Moslem (Qur'an and Hadith).

THE HUMAN RIGHTS OF THE PERSON WITH INTELLECTUAL DISABILITY IN ISLAM

Human Rights, in Islam, are incorporated in the Qur'an, which the Prophet Mohammad received from God. So, these rights should be respected as eternal laws of humankind. Therefore, every Muslim will have to accept, recognize and enforce these human rights. "Those who do not judge by what God has sent down are the disbelievers" (Human Rights in Islam, 1999).

The phrase mentioned earlier: "Nor take life, which God has made sacred except for a just cause," (The Qur'an, Surah Bani Israil 17:33), gives the human fetus the right to exist, to live and to develop and, thus, directly or indirectly nothing is to be done to prevent it from prospering. The Prophet Mohammad said: "This human being is a building of God on this earth and God is going to destroy anyone who is going to destroy this building."

In Islam, children have an important role and honored place in the society. God said in the Qur'an: "We have indeed honored the children of Adam, and have provided for them means of transportation on land and sea, and given them wholesome food, and exalted them high above the greater part of Our creation." This verse shows that each person, irrespective of his race, color, religion or other means of material or mental ability or gender, deserves regard and respect.

According to Prophets' sayings (Hadith): "That person is not one of us, who is not merciful to our juniors and respectful to our olders." People who treat them kindly are promised to visit paradise. Parents and children are commanded to respect each other. This is a clear message of God in the Qur'an and the speech of the Prophet.

In Islam the parent is commanded to have a role in crystalizing good qualities in the child. The child in Islam has the right of having a father (in some cases adopted by a father or by society) and rejects the fact that children may be fatherless. Thus, the father, who is not biological, should be responsible for the material and social support of the child and, for this, he will receive Islamic compassion. Islam recognizes the right of the children to have equal life chances regardless of sex or disability and a parent unrecognizng of this equality is accused of commiting injustice. One Qur'anic verse tells us: "O believers, be you securers of justice, witness for God. Let not detestation for a people move you not to be equitable. Be equitable, that is nearer to God-fearing." There is no permission for opressing women, children, old people the sick, and the wounded. Women's honor and chastity are to be respected, the hungry to be fed, and wounded or diseased to be treated irrespective of being Moslems or not, enemy or friends. Islam also recognizes other human rights, for example; the right to basic necessities of life of the needy and their right for help and assistance to be provided to them: "And in their wealth there is acknowledged right for the needy and the destitute" (Human Rights in Islam, 1999).

In Islam there is the right of the person not to be arrested or imprisoned for the offenses of others. The Holy Qur'an clarifies this issue:

No bearer of burdens shall be made to bear the burden of another. (Qur'an)

The protection of honor is another right of mankind and the Qur'an says: "You who believe, do not let one (set of) people make fun of another set. . . . Do not defame one another. . . . Do not insult by using nicknames." Privacy and security of private life has to be protected, and the Qur'anic verse tells us: "Do not enter any houses unless you are sure of their occupant's consent."

According to Fiqh (Muchtar, 1995), the intellectually disabled are diagnosed as being such by experts, and whenever a person is found to be disabled he is not responsible for his speech and action. According to Islam, the intellectually disabled are eligible for marriage and heritage, but his behavior and decision-making is to be supervised by his guardian. The father of the disabled is his guardian and, if he has died, the grandfather, the uncle or the older brother or the governor (the state) must take upon themselves the responsibility.

Residential care for disabled is not forbidden in Islamic society and such an institution could be the guardian of the disabled, if his family is unable. But if there is a guardian, the institution should provide only for his health and well-being, whereas the guardian is responsible for legal aspects.

HISTORY OF THE CARE OF PERSONS WITH INTELLECTUAL DISABILITY IN ISLAM

In 706, the Caliph Al-Walid Ben Abed Al-Malik permitted the establishment of the first Islamic hospital and declared the medical profession official (Nader, 1995). He ordered, also, the assignment of a caregiver for each disabled and needy person, and permitted an allowance from the imperial treasure for these workers (Nader, 1995).

Khalid Ibn Yazid (end of the 7th century), gave up his wealth for the study of medicine and chemistry. One anecodote from the first years of Islam shows the interest and understanding of the Moslem society for the needs of the disabled. One person complained to the Caliph Omar Ibn Al-Khatab that his son was physically disabled and unable to reach the mosque. The Caliph ordered his subordinates to arrange a closer shelter to the mosque for this disabled person (Anwar, 1973).

By the ninth century Islamic medical practice had reached great advance. From talisman and theology to hospitals and wards of those afflicted with fever, the insane were treated with gentleness, and pain was relieved by walking in gardens, parks and listening to music and story telling. The prince and the poor man received equal medical attention. Hospitals were crowded by patients and staff of both sexes. Permanent and mobile clinics provided care for the disabled and other sufferers (Anwar, 1973).

Medical licensing became a central issue and patient education and legal measures were taken to protect the patients and the rights of the disabled. The famous Islamic physician, Ibn Sinna, known to the West of the medieval period as Avicennum, allocated a great deal of his knowledge to this topic of health of the disabled and practiced psychotherapy. He made great efforts to develop healthy lifestyles for the patient and disabled (Islam, 1973).

In the year 1500, the Islamic physician Al-Hafez published his book on disabilities in an encyclopedic fashion including details on different disabilities in a special scientific classification (Anwar, 1973).

THE SERVICE FOR PERSONS
WITH INTELLECTUAL DISABILITY

Egypt was the first Arab state to pay attention, officially, to the disabled and their needs by allocating three classes at elementary schools for the disabled in 1955 (Nader, 1995). In 1965, this number reached a total of twenty and four institutions were providing care to this population.

In Kuwait two centers were built in 1960 to provide care for the population of persons with intellectual disabilities. One provided care of males and the other to females. In 1965 a center for severly intellectually disabled persons was established (Nader, 1995).

In Syria and Lebanon, the initiative to establish two facilities for persons with intellectual disabilities was taken by in each country in 1960 (Nader, 1995).

Jordan joined this experience for the first time in 1967, when Christian and civil Islamic organizations initiated the movement to establish institutions for the disabled. The Ministry of Social Welfare also participated in opening a number of centers for the intellectually disabled, including the Al-Manar center in Amman, during 1977 (Nader, 1995).

In Israel, the first residential centers for Arabs with intellectual disabilities were established in 1973, and two of them were run by a Christian religious organization and the other by a non-for-profit organization. Today there are 12 centers out of 53 in Israel (23% of the Israeli centers), with a total population of 782 Persons (13% of the population of persons with intellectual disability in residential centers). The centers for Arabs are either privately or publicly administrated, but supported by the Ministry of Labour and Social Affairs, who provides the budget and supervision.

CONCLUSION

This study emphasizes the continuity between the modern and the original historical attitudes of Islam regarding the care for the disabled. This care is justified in the humanistic philosophy of the Islam and founded in the Qur'an and the Islamic theology.

Caring for the disabled is the duty of every Moslem and every Islamic state and society. Empathy, human rights protection and holisitic care for this population deserves a social and economic investment.

The Arab world and Arab communities have the duty to continue with this heritage, to strengthen and enrich this tradition.

REFERENCES

Anwar, A. (1973). *The history of science in Islam.*(Arabic). Beirut, Lebanon: Dar Alfikr.

Human Rights in Islam (1999). <www.unn.ac.uk/societies/islamic/about/islam/07.htm>

Mahmoud, A. (1990). *Sport and welfare for the disabled.* (Arabic). Cairo, Egypt: Maktabat Alnahda Al-misrya.

Muchtar, S. (1995). *The medical creative activity of the Prophet of humanity.* (Arabic). Beirut, Lebanon: Al-Maarif.

Nader, A. (1995). *Teaching the disabled children.* (Arabic). Jordan: Dar Alfekr.

Disabled Women in Islam:
Middle Eastern Perspective

Majid Turmusani, PhD

SUMMARY. Western debates have increasingly included women issues in their analysis. These debates however, proved to have little relevance to women with impairments and are in fact being held under
scrutiny by feminist writers. The position of disabled women in other cultures remains especially one of the most under-researched areas within
current discourses on women and disability issues. This presentation fills
the gap and presents an account based on textual analysis of disabled
women in Islam and Muslim culture. It argues that disabled women in Islam have a lowly position in society due to historical perception related to
both the inferior position of women in Islam as well as the lowly position
of disabled people in society in general. Understanding the position of disabled women thus requires close investigation into these two positions
within their particular socio-economic and historical contexts. Despite the
presence of various feminists' movements in Muslim countries these days,
these have not included much debate on disability and disabled women

---

Majid Turmusani specialises in disability and development and is currently based in
Kosovo with Handicap International working on disability policy and strategy under
the United Nations Mission. After completion of his PhD in 1999, he joined Centre for
International Child Health (CICH), University College London working in a joint CBR
project between WHO and CICH.
Address correspondence to: Dr. Majid Turmusani, People Potential, Plum Cottage,
Hattingley Road, Medstead, Alton, Hampshire, Gu34 5NQ UK (E-mail: turm
usani@hotmail.com).

[Haworth co-indexing entry note]: "Disabled Women in Islam: Middle Eastern Perspective." Turmusani,
Majid. Co-published simultaneously in *Journal of Religion, Disability & Health* (The Haworth Pastoral Press,
an imprint of The Haworth Press, Inc.) Vol. 5, No. 2/3, 2001, pp. 73-85; and: *Spirituality and Intellectual Disability: International Perspectives on the Effect of Culture and Religion on Healing Body, Mind, and Soul*
(eds: William C. Gaventa, Jr. and David L. Coulter) The Haworth Pastoral Press, an imprint of The Haworth
Press, Inc., 2001, pp. 73-85. Single or multiple copies of this article are available for a fee from The Haworth
Document Delivery Service [1-800-342-9678, 9:00 a.m. - 5:00 p.m. (EST). E-mail address:
getinfo@haworthpressinc.com].

within their mainstream analysis.

The paper concludes by calling for existing theoretical perspectives to include the analysis of disabled women within their remit and also to take note of wider contextual issues including cultures, religions, and economy when studying women in society. *[Article copies available for a fee from The Haworth Document Delivery Service: 1-800-342-9678. E-mail address: <getinfo@haworthpressinc.com> Website: <http://www.HaworthPress.com> © 2001 by The Haworth Press, Inc. All rights reserved.]*

KEYWORDS. Islam, disabled women, disabled people, Middle East, Islamic texts, contemporary society, patriarchy, human rights, less (inferior), attitudes, honor killing, economy, ableism [1]

DISABILITY IN THE MIDDLE EAST

Disability in the Middle East is often perceived as divine intervention or work of evil spirit (Jinn) (Miles, 1995; Coleridge, 1999; Habib, 1997), implying impurity and indifference on the part of people who have impairments. In the long run those with impairments are made to feel less than others. The birth of disabled child brings shame and blame to family members especially mothers. These perceptions lead to negative attitudes towards disabled people and results in isolation and invisibility of the person who has impairment. This is an ongoing process and has roots in social and cultural responses to disability.

The previous situation means that the majority of disabled people living in the Middle East are experiencing social and economic deprivation in their life. They have substantially restricted access to services such as education medical care, training, welfare and employment and also are highly represented among the poor in society. The needs of disabled people remain largely unmet. Their life opportunities are restricted and the rights for equality in society go unrecognised.

Traditionally, care for disabled people in the Middle East was provided within the context of home. Typically, the father or able-bodied male members rule family life and disabled people usually have less power over decisions pertaining their lives. This lack of autonomy is especially manifested in the outdoor mobility of disabled women (evidence from Jordan and Lebanon[2]). All too often, women with impairments end up hidden at home as dependent, adjacent on family resources, or in a residential institution away from sight.

When out of the home, the mode of care for disabled people follows charitable institutions. Those with severe impairments are often catered for in residential units.[3] External forces, such as international NGO's, encouraged this trend of care. UN agencies in the region such as UNRWA, the principal UN body created to cater for the needs of Palestinians refugees in the region, for example, focused on emergency relief work rather than sustainable development, as did many international NGO's. Institutional charitable care led to disability being looked at as marginal issue on the political agenda instead of an issue of human rights.

While this is the general trend in viewing disabled people throughout the region, recent years have witnessed a positive change in perception relating to the causes of impairment. In Palestine, for example, men who acquired impairments during Intifada became local heroes and figures in their communities (Habib, 1997). Therefore, it can be argued that, although political conflicts in the Middle East have greatly increased the number of disabled people, these have also led to changes in attitudes towards people with impairments and affected the provision of services.

This change of attitudes, however, was not extended to disabled women. Social responses and parental practices continue to enhance feelings of inferiority on the part of disabled people in general and this becomes especially evident when the disabled person is a female. In times of scarcity of resources, household practices tend to discriminate against disabled female members when allocating resources for instance for education, health care etc. Examples of discriminative parental practices are prevalent throughout the region and empirical evidence of such practices is reported especially from Lebanon and Jordan (Turmusani, 1999).

Disabled people have significantly less chance to get married compared with their counterparts. It is easier, however, for a disabled male to be found in marital relationship than a disabled female. Marriage chances are profoundly affected by the presence of impairments for disabled women because much emphasis is placed on the physical ability of women to cater for household in the Middle East. The lives of those unmarried women are often regarded as not worth living. This widely held belief is endorsed not only by culture but also by Islamic traditions towards the notion of *ableisim* and gender roles as will be explained later on. Moreover, disabled women are twice as prone to divorce, separation and violence as able-bodied women (DAA/UNESCO, 1995). The frequent exclusion of disabled women from rehabilitation programs in the Middle East (Coleridge, 1993) means that these meet only the needs of disabled men, helping them to recover their masculinity and sexuality (Begum, 1992; Morris, 1993).

In conclusion to this section, Islamic values, still dominant in the Middle East, regulate the position of women in society and apply equally to women with impairments. These cultural norms are based on textual evidence deriving from major sources, which makes them powerful and relevant to people's lives. The way in which these values are constructed in the texts and how they affect disabled women will be explored next.

ISLAMIC TEXTS [4] AND DISABLED WOMEN

Generally speaking, disability in a man's family was often concealed in Islamic society and women tended to be kept out of public eyes. Women with impairments were especially made invisible in traditional Muslim society.

Islamic society is organised and maintained by a set of teachings and principles deriving chiefly from Qur'an and Hadith[5]. Everything revolves around one powerful character called "Allah" or God. The image of this God in Islam refers to "He" an extension of patriarchal power. This image is perfect in power as well as the physical character (see, hear, walk, etc.). For those who can't see, hear, walk, etc., (i.e., disabled) they break the notion of normalcy and are regarded as different.

It is stated that in Islam men are superior to women and women must accept men's authority and obey their commands. This makes it clear that Islam is strictly patriarchal society and explicitly internalises male dominance or what is being referred to in Qur'an as "Qawwamun" (2:228). This concept for Ibn Kathir means men are 'the boss,' have authority and can discipline women. They are superior for two reasons, first, for their mental and physical capabilities and, second, for their responsibility to maintain women financially (Ibn Kathir, 1996).

Men's extra rights and superiority can be seen in Qur'anic texts in their power to divorce (2:231); polygamy (4:3); advantages in inheritance (4:11); and the right to take extreme measures in disciplining women such as enforcing Hijab (24:31) on them and beating them (4:34). Women are also in an inferior position when compared to men in regard to their chances to pursue economic and political activities. For example, in business transactions women need 2 witnesses instead of one as is the case with men. This ratio of 2/1 female to male witnesses is applied not only in business but also in all spheres of life.

Women in Hadith are referred to as those created for men's comfort and merely as a vessel of procreation (2:233). At the spiritual level women are portrayed as less spiritual beings, as mentioned above, due to lack of religion (1:142) and subsequently not allowed to take part in spiritual leadership roles such as Imam. [6] Moreover, women are not encouraged to be rulers (Ibn Kathir, Hadith). There has been no position of Imam ever occupied by a woman throughout Islamic history. Generally speaking, women are being held responsible for the downfall of humanity, lacking spiritual materials and often referred to as harmful to man (36:6603) and as having an evil omen (62:30). Constantly, women are mentioned in Hadith as residents of hell Book (24:5310).

Despite the improved position of women in Islamic Middle Eastern society, they are still regarded as "awra," which means that a woman's face and body must not be exposed to public view and, also that their life chances are restricted by the decisions of men (Turmusani, 1999). This is how the tradition of women wearing "Hijab" came about in Islamic society following the endorsement of Hijab by Qur'an and Hadith.

Like women, disabled people are also disadvantaged in their lives within Muslim culture. Islamic texts have generally portrayed people with impairments as less and as different. Various references in the book portray people with impairments in rather negative ways, associating them with evil-doers, unbelievers, and even beasts (Anfal, 8:22), and others (Turmusani, 1999). Icons of Islamic enemies, for example, are repeatedly portrayed with physical disfigurements. Book (37:4306) in Hadith describes those who will loot the holy place in Mecca as having short legs. Al-dajal (the Antichrist) is also described as being a short man with one eye. Such representation, it is argued, has served to perpetuate societal negative attitudes and discriminative practices towards disabled people.

While only blind people have been referred to in some positive sense in Qur'an and Hadith, there are various statements referring to other types of impairments in a negative and stigmatic way. Book (56:670) describes lepers and people with baldness as unhelpful and unfaithful to favour. Book (23:3994) similarly portrays those with weak intellect as being devious. Hadith goes further in mistrusting the abilities of people with impairments, suggesting no hope for those people becoming contributing members of society. Book (1:6) for example, gives a sign of end of days as the time when deaf and dumb people become able to take part in public affairs.

In brief, both women and disabled people in Islam experience oppression and discrimination as disadvantaged groups in society–a society that is designed for the able-bodied male. This position is perpetuated by the negative representation of disabled people in various Islamic texts. Qur'anic materials make clear distinctions between ablesim and disabilism. The notion of ableism can be seen in a number of verses, but most notably in Al-An'am (6:50), Hud (11:24), the Angles (35:19) and the Believer (40:58). Here, people who have impairments are presented as unequal and as less to those who do not have impairments in their bodies or mind.

Overall, there are only few incidents in Islamic texts (Qur'an and Hadith) that refer to women with impairments. Those texts make negative references to disabled people in general compounding negative views of women with impairments. For example, in Isra' (17:97) and Ta-ha (20:124), unbelievers will be raised on the day of judgement with various impairments such as blindness, deafness, dumbness, etc., and will abide hell. This applies to both men and women. Although, there is no direct Qur'anic reference to women with impairments, a number of Hadith texts refer to women residing in hell as having physical disfigurement in their heads (Book 36:6596).

It is argued that this negative representation of disabled women in Islamic texts has contributed to their inferior position in society. Because they were perceived by society as 'less' and as 'others' negative attitudes were generated towards them and few provisions were made in their favour. Over time, inferiority of disabled women became the norm in society and issues of their equality and human rights were rarely discussed in debates and policy agenda until recently.

DISABLING PRACTICES AGAINST DISABLED WOMEN IN CONTEMPORARY ISLAMIC SOCIETY

Disabling practices against disabled women in the Middle Eastern culture are manifested in everyday life experience. For the majority of disabled women, this means restricted access or no access to services such as education, health care, training, employment, etc. This discrimination, as mentioned previously, has roots in social and cultural responses to disability and is endorsed by Islamic teachings.

Neglect and abuse of disabled women continue to exist in the Middle East while no debate has taken place over these issues until recently. Such abuse has roots in household practices and includes females in different age groups. Despite recent developments in disability services in the region, disabled women are still disadvantaged in a variety of ways. Recent incidence of parental abuse of disabled women is reported from Jordan for example (DAA, 2000). The Finnish Government has protested against the very poor living condition of disabled children in a refugee camp in Jordan. The background of this case is that two children were placed in foster care in Denmark after reported abuse by their natural parents. This year however, Copenhagen Council's decision ruled to remove the disabled children from their foster parents and return them to their natural parents in Jordan.

In Lebanon, this goes even further: a father left his disabled daughter open to the risk of dying in their half-destroyed house in South Lebanon after Israeli offensive struck the village. He chose to salvage the cow instead because it was more useful (Habib, 1997).

In Palestine, honour killing, a widespread practice,[7] was also extended to a disabled woman with visible "mental retardation." Although she was raped and assaulted by her attacker, the death penalty had to be carried out and her relatives had her killed in accordance with honour killing practices in Muslim culture.

Empirical evidence from Jordan suggests that the lowly position of women in Islamic society is clearly manifested in women with impairments. Views from those interviewed within the course of research on the economic needs of disabled people confirm such a claim (Turmusani, 1999 [8]). Participants have often internalised a feeling of inferiority and accepted male dominance in their lives in accordance with dominant Islamic norms. For example, some of them expressed their dissatisfaction about the limited job opportunities available in the labour market and how this impacted their lives and their autonomy. However, when they were asked whether they should have equal access to those limited jobs, they often gave priority to their disabled male counterparts.

Disabled women also internalised views towards their family life as living single and as dependent on other male members of their families. Those residing in institutions were more likely to accept passive role in their lives and let male members decide on their behalf concerning education, training, etc. Educated women with mild impairments however, were more assertive in their views for rights to establish family and access to services in general.

Other examples included parental practices towards disabled family members, which give preference to disabled males in access to services as mentioned previously. When more than one case of impairment exist within the family, female members were often placed in residential units, whereas male members were allowed admission to daily care centers and continued to have physical presence in family life.

As argued earlier, women and disabled women in Islam are particularly restricted in pursuing economic activities such as establishing business. Generally there are limited credit facilities available that include disabled people in their services. The ones that exist require complicated procedures and collateral that the majority of disabled women usually cannot afford. Cultural attitudes towards women's abilities and their outdoor mobility further restrict their chances to engage in the economy. Islamic traditions request women to seek men's concession before embarking on major projects such as running a business. Evidence from Jordan shows that women, including disabled women, are required to obtain their husbands' permission before they are allowed credit for their business.

It can be concluded that in business as in other areas of life, the general public attitudes towards disabled women's ability and the restrictions imposed on their outdoor mobility are determinant factors for inclusion in society. Those who run their own businesses in Jordan, for example, have reported the lack of family support and negative public attitudes towards them as major obstacles in successful business enterprises. Women and disabled women in Islamic society are viewed as 'less' than men and, as such, are left under their guardianship. This perception has roots in family's up-bringing practices as pointed out earlier.

FEMINISTS' PERSPECTIVE ON DISABILITY IN THE MIDDLE EAST

Current feminist rhetoric had often failed to address the issue of women with disabilities and the marginalization of their interests and contribution to development (Sen, 1995). Until recently, in Islamic society of the Middle East, disabled women have received little attention from women's movements, if at all. This is not surprising given that these movements are quite new to the region and are busy trying to lay down the foundation of the work in such hostile environments. Moreover, these movements are also engaged in issues concerning access to services such as education, employment, etc. That said, it should be noted that even in the West, disabled women's issues are still alienated from disability movement's discourse (Morris, 1996; Crow, 1996). These writers, along with others, argue that the disability movement, notably in the UK, is dominated by male disabled theorists and to a large extent excludes disabled women. Moreover, there is little manifestation of disabled women's experience of body and pain in their analysis of disability.

Feminism is defined as an individual or collective awareness recognizing that women have been and continue to be oppressed in diverse ways and for diverse reasons because of gender. Feminism aims towards liberation from oppression and calls for a more equitable society with improved relations between men and women (Nicholson and Fraser, 1990). Feminism, in this sense, bears similarity with other social movements such as disabled people movements and the black movement, which all strive to overcome the cause–the roots of oppression and dis-empowerment.

The term "feminism" originated in the west and was introduced to the Arab Muslim countries in the post-colonial era. In the Middle East, it is characterised as being 'western' and a 'bad thing' and as a strategic colonial technique to undermine the order of social and religious culture. It is full of negative stereotypes, for example, feminism is often presented by religious leaders as a western attack on Islam as oppressive and backward.

There are different kinds of feminists groups in the Middle East including Islamists, Muslims and seculars and are mentioned briefly. Islamists feminists are part of political movement that is on the whole actively attempting to raise support for itself in its ultimate quest for the capture of state power and legislation. Muslim feminists on the other hand are more likely to form part of more mainstream women's groups. Like secular feminists they lack the support of the state. While Muslim feminists trying to reconcile the discourses of Islam with human rights, they both face the same accusation of being culturally inauthentic secular feminists. Secular feminists place their argument out of religious groups into the human rights perspective. Religion is a private matter that should not form any political agenda (El Saadawi, 1997).

There are various forces, which undermine feminists' progress in the Middle East. Among them is the dominant Islamic mainstream thought, which endorses a perspective that feminism is irrelevant to Islamic society. The current debate on women issues in the region nonetheless, concerns issues of equity–women's access to rights–rather than equality.

Islamic values thus continue to influence feminists thinking and to a large extent determine their agenda. This is despite the active presence of women in NGO's (charities) and humanitarian aid agencies for decades since the second half of last century. In the Middle East, it is argued that a movement such as feminism, which does not justify itself within Islam, is bound to be rejected by the rest of Muslim society.

Only secular feminists groups have some autonomy in expressing radical views towards women's issues in Muslim culture. Their impact to influence political agendas, however, remains limited as mentioned above. Reinforced by international pressure, secular feminists did make exceptions in the Middle East though. For example, in Jordan feminists lobbies backed up by international support led to changes in legislation to ban widespread practice of honour killing. Although in practice, this was only endorsed on paper, it is nevertheless considerable progress on this front.

In contrast, feminist's lobbies in Egypt have almost failed to make a substantial difference regarding contemporary issues such as Female Genital Mutilation (FGM). The general modes in society continue to vote in favour of Islamic views towards these practices and feminists rhetoric on this issue continue to be neglected (http://www.geocities. com/~lrrc/FGM/fgm.htm).

To conclude, feminists in the Middle East, generally speaking, have failed to take note of disabled women's issues in their mainstream analysis. As argued above, they have been engaged in other pressing issues such as poverty among women, unemployment and access to services and therefore, disabled women issues do not appear as priority. When they do discuss issues pertinent to women with disabilities however, this usually occurs as part of the wider debate on women.

TOWARDS INCLUSIVE ANALYSIS

Despite the dominance of Islamic culture in Middle East, variations and particularities exist between countries as well as between regions. Disparity can be found even within one single country and the obvious example is Israel with three main religions, two or more languages and varying levels of advancement and technology. Historically, this region has always been under the rule of foreign nations and only recently has become independent from Western colonization. Previous variation means that disability has been understood and dealt with differently.

Contemporarily, this region has witnessed hot politics and is characterized as one of the most volatile places in the world. The historical, religious and strategic value of the Middle East meant that extensive international efforts are being made to bring peace and harmony into the region. Besides imported Western technologies, western debates are also extended to the local scene. Among those introduced were social movements such as women's and disabled people's movements. These debates however, remain limited in scope and their influence over public agenda.

Both idealists and materialist approaches to social change are Western created notions. These argue that scientific engagement in debating social issues can materialize in bringing the aspired change in society. Academic and advocate discourses are essential means in this process. Black and disabled people's movements are but few examples.

Theoretical debates have potential impact far beyond the academic circle into the life of the community. Changing the position of disabled women through debate in the Middle East, however, has proved to be limited so far. This might be attributed to the prominence of other traditional vehicles used for social change in this region. The perception of women issues as low priority by society often lead to these issues being excluded from mainstream debate and subsequent policies.

This paper suggests, in brief, that the position of disabled women in Islamic society can substantially be improved by drawing on the strength and resources of other existing groups such as feminists groups and the growing lobby of disabled people. It is crucial that various debates in society take note of disabled women's issues in their analysis. Debate should ultimately aim at fighting the negative representation of disabled women within culture and society.

CONCLUSION

This account primarily explored the position of disabled women in Islamic society and how socio-economic and historical factors affected disabled women in contemporary Middle Eastern culture. It is argued that the negative representation of women and disabled people in Islamic texts has led to their inferior position in society. Discrimination against women including those with impairments in Islam compounds the oppression theory to women with disabilities in general.

While physical and sexual abuse of disabled women occurs in the Middle East, there have been no debates or recognition of such a problem until now. This is attributed to the Islamic approach in dealing with social problems by hiding them in an attempt to keep society intact and protected. Feminist debate on this front has been limited mainly to women's issues in general and not disabled women. Their arguments are constantly neglected and rejected by a more powerful Islamic thinking in contemporary Middle Eastern culture.

It is hoped that by changing the interpretations of how disabled women are represented in Islamic texts through current debates we can substantially change the status and position of disabled women in society.

NOTES

1. Ableism in the UK refers to the notion of 'normalcy, normal, etc.' Also the use of the term 'disabled person" is widely used in the UK as preferable to 'people first' language. It is considered part of a person's identity and nothing to be hidden.

2. Examples include restrictions on decisions pertaining to life such as undertaking education, employment and wider relationships with others (Habib, 1997, Turmusani, 1999).

3. In Jordan, for example, a specialised unit was established with Saudi and UN sponsorship to provide residential services for blind women. Many residents in this institution have reported being left too long without going home or being visited by family members (Turmusani, 1999).

4. Islamic texts here refer mainly to Qur'an and Hadith, which are cited in the list of bibliography. Hadith materials were found when surfing the web, end of September 2000 at the following site: <http://islam.org/mosque/surai.htm> Same URL contains a directory of Qur'anic text with web search facility.

5. Hadith refer to what Mohammed did or said during his prophetic life. Hadith text is arranged into smaller sections known as Book/s.

6. Western Feminists argue that the patriarchal image of God within main world religions has contributed to women oppression in general. In Islamic context however, while spiritual work continues to be limited to men only, in Christianity for example, women succeeded to become priests and other spiritual activities. This however, is not meant to argue the preference and advantages of one religion over the other.

7. "Honour Killing" refers to practices of killing female relatives who are caught in immoral sexual behaviours by family male members. This is a widespread practice until today and is endorsed by some Islamic traditions related to measures dealing with adultery and women in general. Honour killing is also prominent in other Islamic countries such as Pakistan (Coleridge, 2000).

8. This concerns an empirical research carried out to investigate the economic needs of disabled men and women in Jordan during 1996 and completed in 1999.

REFERENCES

Ali, A (1991) The Meaning of the Holy Qur'an (transl.). Maryland: Ammana Corporation, Brentwood.

Begum, N (1992) Disabled Women and the Feminist Agenda. *Feminist Review*, No 40, 1992.

Coleridge, P (2000) Culture and Disability. Asian Pacific Disability and Rehabilitation Journal: Selected readings in CBR. January 2000-09-14.

Crow, L (1993) Including All of Our Lives: Renewing the social model of disability. In Barnes, C & Mercer, G (Eds.) Exploring the Divide: Illness and disability. Leeds: The Disability Press.

DAA (2000) Exporting "Problem" Children from Denmark. Disability Tribune; The International Disability and Human Rights Network. March 2000.

DAA/UNESCO (1995) Overcoming Obstacles to the Integration of Disabled people. Copenhagen.

Habib, L (1997) Gender and Disability: Women experiences in the Middle East. London: Oxfam.

Ibn Kathir (1996) Tafsir Al Qur'an Al-A'dim (2nd ed., Vol. 1, 1996).

Khan, M (1979) The Translation of the meaning of Sahih Al Bukhari, Arabic-English. Vol. VIII. Chicago: Kazi.

Lang, R (2000) The Role of NGO's in the Process of Empowerment and Social Transformation of People with Disabilities. *Asia Pacific Disability Rehabilitation Journal: Selected readings in community based rehabilitation.* Series 1, CBR in Transition, 2000.

Miles, M (1995) Disability within Eastern Religious Context. *Disability and Society*, Vol. 10 (1), 1995.

Morris, J. (1996) Encounter with Strangers: Feminism and disability. London: The Women's Press.

Nicholson, L & Fraser N (1990) Social Criticism without Philosophy: An encounter between Feminism and Postmodernism. In Nicholson, L (Ed.) Feminism/Postmodernism. London and New York: Routledge.

Saadawi, N (1997) The Nawal El Saadawi Reader. London: Zed Books.

Sen, K (1995) Gender, Culture and Later Life: A dilemma for contemporary feminism. *Gender and Development*, Vol. 3 (3) 1995.

Shakespeare, T. (1994) Cultural Representation of Disabled People: Dustbin for disavowal? *Disability and Society*, 9, (3) 283-299.

Turmusani, M (1999) Some Cultural Representation of Disabled People in Jordan: Concepts and beliefs. In Holzer B et al (Eds.) Disability in Different Cultures: Reflections on local concepts. Beilefeld, Germany: Verlag Muhlenstrabe.

Cultural/Spiritual Attributions as Independent Variables in the Development of Identity and Potential for Persons of Exceptionality: A Case Study of North American Christianity and Native American Religious Influence

Candace Cole-McCrea, MA, PhD (candidate)

SUMMARY. In Anglo social and religious culture, personal biological characteristics of exceptionality result in social attributions of inferiority, reduced social responsibility and reduced status. In Native American social and religious culture, these same personal characteristics result in social attributions and expectations of extraordinary ability, increased social responsibility, and honored status. A principle shared by both, however, is that the Life experience of each person can be a Divine Calling. Religious and socio-cultural attributions operate as independent variables of socialization asserting far stronger effects upon the real life outcomes of human exceptionality than biology ever may. Assumptions

---

Candace Cole-McCrea is Chair, Department of Human Services and Social Sciences, New Hampshire Community Technical College, Stratham, New Hampshire, P.O. Box 1033, Milton, NH 03851-1033 (E-mail: snowyowl@ usadatanet.net).

[Haworth co-indexing entry note]: "Cultural/Spiritual Attributions as Independent Variables in the Development of Identity and Potential for Persons of Exceptionality: A Case Study of North American Christianity and Native American Religious Influence." Cole-McCrea, Candace. Co-published simultaneously in *Journal of Religion, Disability & Health* (The Haworth Pastoral Press, an imprint of The Haworth Press, Inc.) Vol. 5, No. 2/3, 2001, pp. 87-98; and: *Spirituality and Intellectual Disability: International Perspectives on the Effect of Culture and Religion on Healing Body, Mind, and Soul* (eds: William C. Gaventa Jr. and David L. Coulter) The Haworth Pastoral Press, an imprint of The Haworth Press, Inc., 2001, pp. 87-98. Single or multiple copies of this article are available for a fee from The Haworth Document Delivery Service [1-800-342-9678, 9:00 a.m. - 5:00 p.m. (EST). E-mail address: getinfo@haworthpressinc.com].

of Selfhood and of exceptionality within Native American Spirituality and North American Christianity are compared and contrasted, proposing an analysis using the bell curve in an unorthodox manner to unify both perspectives. Specific examples are drawn from the author's own experience as a full professor and academic chair, psychologist, minister, elder and seer of Mohawk Native American ancestry, and as a person who grew up as a retarded, severely multiply disabled child receiving the socialization of both cultures and belief systems. The author concludes with a proposal that we return to the shared principle of each culture: that the life experience of each person can be a Divine Calling. This principle is illustrated through her successful interventions with severely disabled children, one of whom she has adopted. It is suggested that we do not use our religions, our sciences, our belief systems, our cultures, as weapons of reductionistic authoritarianism that diminish the quality and potential of any human life. *[Article copies available for a fee from The Haworth Document Delivery Service: 1-800-342-9678. E-mail address: <getinfo@haworthpressinc.com> Website: <http://www.HaworthPress.com> © 2001 by The Haworth Press, Inc. All rights reserved.]*

KEYWORDS. Native American, calling, spirituality, disability

In 1994, I took in a special needs foster child. He was 10 days old and was abandoned in an inner city in the cold, New Hampshire March weather. Social Services brought him to me because of my specialty in terminal or severely ill infants and also because he was Native American, as am I. This infant was premature, had failure to thrive syndrome, and was born addicted to heroin, cocaine, alcohol and nicotine. His mother was HIV positive and so he also tested positive, carrying her antibodies. His mother had also consumed drugs during the week after his birth and had nursed him with her drugged milk before she abandoned him. I took a year off work immediately to care for him. I carried him in a pouch for his entire first year, except when I took a shower, which I only did if someone else could hold him. He went into seizures; he became semi-comatose, shutting out the world around him. He vomited everything I fed him (until I discovered that if I hummed to him while I fed him and, for a while thereafter, he could digest his food). He shook with cold incessantly; he stopped breathing often; and his cry was the weakest, saddest cry I had ever heard.

I carried him in a pouch close to my body for one full year; he even slept the night upon my belly as I lay on my back, supporting him. When he started to demise, I had to be able to respond immediately. During that first year, he never babbled; he never learned to sit up, to play with his feet, to do all those ordinary developmental tasks that infants do. Professionals said he was retarded and they wanted to start Early Intervention. I refused and they backed away, since they had no one else who would take care of such a sick and stigmatized Native American infant. I searched and found a well respected physician who also believed in the innate potential in every life. I carefully chose who this child was in the company of; while I did not limit him to being with Native Americans, I was very particular that he would only see, feel, hear of his worth and great potential.

In his second year, his self was strong enough that I was able to move him into a tiny, newborn crib, right next to my bed, and whenever his respiration started to change into a weakening spiral, I only needed to reach over and rub his back and speak to him. I did not need to hold him any longer to carry him through these crises. With my touch and words, he could pull himself through. In the third year, I moved him to a regular sized crib on the other side of my bedroom. When his breathing would change, I needed only to speak and not to touch him at all. In his fourth year, I moved him to his own bedroom and he has not suffered so since.

He did not sit up until he was over a year old. He did not play with infant toys. He whined, he cried, and he lay listlessly still. But, he responded, always, every waking moment, by keeping his eyes upon me. And when I spoke to him, he never failed to calm, no matter how severe the seizures, the colic, etc. At eighteen months, he began to self motivate to sit and to stand. Eventually he would walk. At 4 years, he would begin to run.

He never spoke; he never babbled, until one day, at age 2 1/2, as I walked out, ready to go to work, he looked up at me from his seat on the floor and said in perfect English, "You look very pretty today, Marmee." Needless to say, I cried. Today at 6 years old, he talks incessantly, asking me the meaning of words like "conversational," "defensively," "clarity," to name a few that came up this week.

Gratefully, he sero-converted–he is not HIV positive any longer. He is a Fetal Alcohol Syndrome survivor with a characteristic symptomatic history. But today, at age 6, he learns at a second grade level, is articulate, is creative, is a happy child who controls his own behavior and exhibits good pro-social behavior and manners. His mind is exceptional; he is sensitive to others. He is contentedly immersed in Native culture as well as selectively participating in American cultural/social activities. He is home schooled, belongs to a health club and is a member of a Quaker community and will soon begin 4H. This year, he made front page newspaper coverage, as he initiated a challenge to Kellogg's cereal company for their advertising that was irresponsible to the safety needs of children. Yes, there is central nervous system damage but, accommodations are easily made, and he fits in well with any non-aggressive peers. (He does not like hostile, aggressive behavior in anyone and remains very sensitive to this behavioral style).

Given the common experience and prognosis of children born only with FAS, the question arises as to how it is possible that a child could do so well given the teratogenic influences on him from zygote through embryo through neonate development? And how could he do so well given the expectations and prognosis he faced and faces in American society?

*****

I spent my childhood hidden, sometimes going to school, sometimes not, sometimes institutionalized, sometimes not. I was recognized as a retarded, multiply disabled child and, if social identity is Self, so I truly was. I saw myself as nothing more. I remember a conflict around me when I was hospitalized at age 12–some people wondered if I could be capable of learning how to roll balls of yarn, others knew it was not possible. Finally, I was allowed to try. How delighted I was to accomplish something helpful! Professionals were so surprised at my enthusiasm and ability that my story appeared in a national Occupational Therapy publication, concluding that, maybe, other children like myself could do something as well. This was 1960.

Throughout my childhood and early adulthood, I accomplished many things–I taught myself to read; I was very gifted at arts and crafts. However, later I realized that rather than each of these accomplishments leading to a questioning of my labels and potential, in fact, they just added a savant-like connotation.

Yet, today, I chair a Department of Human Services and Social Sciences at a community college. I am a minister, certified in many professional areas, a published poet. I have a jazz band. I am completing a PhD in psychology this year (having walked away in my final year at Boston University to care for the infant mentioned above). I counsel others and serve as a Native American spiritual elder within my community. And, along the way, my IQ went from 77 to 100 to 110 to 135 to 145 to 162 as I became more and more familiar with the western common stock of knowledge!

When I tested for my GRE's, I scored in the 99th percentile on logic/reasoning. How did this happen?

In 1975, in my 27th year, I was homeless in California and heard that there was a new program that helped severely disabled people find jobs. I could not imagine them helping me. I was in a wheelchair much of the time, was retarded, and legally blind. But I went anyway. My interview was with the Handicapped Services director for the program who happened to also be the director of the new office of Handicapped Services at California State University, Fullerton. During our interview, he asked me why I did not go to college. I thought that was the most stupid thing that anyone ever said to me. But, I was hungry. So when he explained that he could get funding to help me live while I went to school, I thought to myself that at least I would be able to eat for a couple of weeks before they discovered that I was not able to do this. So, I lied. I told him that I had a G.E.D. He enrolled me and gave me a tape recorder and multiple other supports. Three and one half years later, I graduated with 2 majors and a minor and a 3.94 average (I did not know enough to drop a course I never attended) and was hired at professional status as I began graduate school. How did this happen?

Of course, there are multiple variables that affect any person at any point in their lives and it is somewhat arbitrary to highlight any one or two and reify them as causal. That is not my purpose; however, even given this qualification, there are still factors that may be significantly worthy of consideration and evaluation. One is the fact that when I enrolled in the university, I checked Native American on the registration form in spite of the fact that I had been raised within a Christian and secular western culture, alienated from my ancestry. This act to acknowledge my ancestry lead to immediate social ramifications as the Native American Studies program director was promptly informed of my presence and a band of native students and faculty sought me out, including me from then on in all of their endeavors. While the college accommodations made it physically possible for me to attend college, this would not have been sufficient for me to transcend my previous identity and become who I am today. Changes in laws and physical structure accommodations are necessary but not sufficient for persons, whether disabled, of minority races, women, etc., to reach their potential, or to even believe they have one. For me, the key was to be immersed in a Native American community wherein my value and potential as a human being were never questioned or doubted. By definition, as a human being, I was seen as gifted, regardless of my physical condition. The question was only: How was I gifted? There was no doubt that I would and could contribute to humanity. That was a given, both because of my human nature and because it is commonly (though not universally) held within Native American circles that the best leaders suffer and transcend inflictions and crises that the common person never is called to face.

Ramps were built, tape recorders and note takers were provided, tutoring support was given and, maybe, with only this, I would have graduated from college, but I would never have become who I am today if I hadn't been included amongst a people who looked me in the eye, who accepted me as a contributing person, who respected my opinion, who taught me that my exceptional history left me with a responsibility for an extraordinary social contribution. I listened to them; I learned; I studied everything I could get my hands on; I believed; eventually, I even saw; and today, I am becoming able to walk.

It has been 20 years since I began college. I have learned that I am highly influenced by social expectations and beliefs. For nearly the first 30 years of my life, I learned from others that I was severely incapable, with no Self of value to anyone (though I was very loved). During the next 20+ years of my life, I learned from others that I was and am extraordinarily capable, with a Self of great value, first, to my communities of heritage, then later generalizing to professional roles and responsibilities within the dominant American culture. I am free.

Today, I turn back to ask, "why?" and, "how?" and, even more significantly, I turn back to ask: how many others face a similar situation?

I am not a cultural determinist. I am also not suggesting that there are not extreme cases wherein organic factors can not be transcended, even to some degree. Of course there are, and increasingly, with the advances in neonate intensive care medicine. I, will, regardless of social or cultural milieu, never be a ballerina, nor six and a half feet tall. I am not arguing that there is not a biological vessel capacity; I am questioning when and how we maximize that very capacity, or even see it, for that matter. I am not arguing that there is no innate level of intelligence; I am questioning when we realize the fluidity of that capacity, and when we do not. We now know that synapses in the brain grow, connect or atrophy dependent upon stimulation. We are learning that we have a much more powerful effect on each other's ability than we ever believed.

Limits of case study analysis, and of anecdotal research are recognized and acknowledged. But to know the limits does not dismiss the fact that case studies open avenues, feeding future research and understanding. Case studies can challenge current thinking. Even without bringing in the myriad other cases I have worked with, it is my hope that this paper accomplishes this task.

This paper supports the radical (in their time and ours) theories of G.H. Mead, Erving Goffman, and Thomas Szasz, each who espoused that Self is a social creation. It also supports the current paradigm shift within secular institutionalized western cultural patterns begun by Wolfensberger who stated that mentally retarded people suffer from a social disorder more than from a personal impairment when they are viewed as "negatively charged" (Wolfensberger 1972, 13). Wolfensberger proposed the institutionalization of normalization and inclusion as a remedy. Many would say that we have had at least moderate success in achieving these goals. People who have disabilities are now more often seen in our communities doing "normal" things. However, I assert that there are significant limits to the positive effectiveness of normalization and inclusion, as practiced within the public domain thus far, and that we have not truly begun to actualize the mandates proscribed by Wolfensberger. We, indeed, may never be able to do so without the concerted efforts of religious institutions of all faiths. As we have discovered in the aftermath of the Civil Rights movement in the United States, we can change the laws . . . we can change the public practices . . . but until we change the mindsets of individuals–their assumptions and rationale for discrimination and exclusion–devaluing will still occur. Herein, I see a vital task for religious bodies, a task that many Native American tribes have historically accomplished through moral tradition, mythology and socialization ethical practices. Herein, many other religions of the world are also seriously lacking, or worse, contributing to the discrimination and devaluing of persons of difference–whatever the difference may be.

Religions of the dominant cultures have, for the most part, failed miserably at socializing normalization, equality and the valuing of all human life. In the United States, where Jewish and Christian beliefs predominate, there is historical tradition to support discrimination and exclusion. Discrimination and exclusion that result in persons with disabilities having to not only resolve internalized judgments regarding their organic/physical limitations, but to also resolve internalized judgements regarding their moral and human worth–and even their conception of themselves in relationship to the Divine (however the Divine is defined).

Deland (1999) interviewed a number of people who have disabilities to reveal how their religious socialization affected their conceptions of themselves as persons with disabilities. She describes people growing up learning that all diseases and disabilities are evil, that God punishes the wicked with suffering, disease and other losses. " . . . The Biblical record which has shaped Judeo-Christian and cultural attitudes towards disease and disability also has helped to marginalize and ostracize people with disabilities. . . . God is imaged as one who sends disease or disability as a punishment or as a test of faith or endurance. The Hebrew Scriptures are replete with examples which would seem to support the notion of a sin/disability causal relationship and reinforce the image of a God of retributive justice" (Deland 1999, 54). Individuals with disabilities are commonly seen in the public eye as inferior beings of no positive value, even to God!

Contrast this with the socialization within many aboriginal Native American cultures wherein it is taken for granted that the most exceptional human beings who will become the leaders and teachers of the tribe will come from amongst those who have learned through facing extreme adversity, limitations or hardship. Native histories are full of the life stories of people who have been severely challenged or impaired, people who have become elders, seers, chiefs, and leaders of their nation. Of course, no one has to achieve such status to be recognized as having value, of being a Valued Self contributing within a community. While it is not taken for granted that every person facing such issues will become a leader or elder of the tribe, it is accepted that everyone, regardless, is designed by the Creator to contribute to society. As Nuttall (1998, 181) who studied the Inuit culture, wrote, "In such a cultural context, people become human beings and participate as social persons despite instances of what, in other cultural contexts, may be defined as intellectual incompetence, mental illness . . . and so on. This is not to deny that Inuit do recognize that there are individuals who are more or less competent, whether socially or intellectually, than others. However, if someone is born deaf and dumb, or has a disability which may inspire feelings of pity in others, they are to be regarded as a person none-the-less; they are included in all aspects of social life, and not excluded because of what is regarded as a state (-neg) rather than a category of person."

It was into such a cultural spiritual belief system that I found myself as I entered the Native American enclave within college. It is into such a cultural spiritual belief system that I raise my young son. He is taught that he is gifted, that he has a responsibility to God, to himself, and to his community to discover his gifts and to contribute them . . . that his personal issues do not take from his gifts, nor from his responsibility. It was not surprising that as a toddler, my son was honored by the elders in a dedication dance at the local Pow-Wow and presented with a blanket. Since then, elders and community members have given him gifts of feathers and other handmade crafts. His Calling, his significance, his value as a human being is reinforced, continuously. Recently, elders were discussing how soon to teach him to drum–a rare honor for one young or old, very rarely considered before adolescence. He is learning his social/spiritual place within community, within his world regardless of his physical history or current central nervous system damage. Is it any wonder, then, that I do not send him to public school, where he would be placed in special education, and learn that he is inferior; or in a Sunday school where he may learn he was not designed by a loving God?

Herein is where we have failed to institute Wolfensberger's conceptions of normalization in our lives and where religions are significantly responsible. (True, education and family institutions are also responsible but the problems within each of these institutions is addressed regularly in the public media today so will not be addressed here). I propose that, while Wolfensberger prescribed that people with disabilities should be integrated into culturally normative settings. He also prescribed that within such settings these same people must be given socially valued roles "to provide the framework for a cathedral of human dignity" (Wolfensberger 1972, 73). I assert that it is this second condition that we have effectively failed to appreciate and, herein, I take religions to task.

What if religions taught, as liberation theology and Native American culture are modeling, that all human life is sacred and that anything sacred must have value; that by definition a spiritual practice does not devalue Life? What if social norms changed within religions such that persons of difference were seen, philosophically, historically, religiously, as persons deserving not only of charity (defined in the modern sense of the word as material help), but also capable of respectful contribution? (I am not talking about just scrubbing the floors here, though, as Gandhi reminded us, that is a significant contribution. I doubt, however, that even he would have liked to have been limited to it.) What if religions recognized that as agents of socialization, they contribute fundamentally to the mindset that becomes self or that sees, allows, creates or destroys self in others? What if I didn't have to wait thirty years to be accepted, valued as a human being? What if no one did?

I have compared and contrasted basic assumptions of personhood, social life, and Divine design for human definition between western religious traditions and Native American spirituality. However, I have left out a fundamental principle found within each that could become a unifying thread for the social betterment of all. Within each there is the principle of a Divine Calling. It is assumed that persons may be Called by the Divine to serve the community in some particular way and that their lives thereafter may be lived to reflect the significance of that Calling. This idea is found in Native American cultures and in western religions. The difference is that in Native American cultures it is commonly held that there exists a Calling for each individual; within western religions, a Calling may only be recognized and sanctioned for an exceptional few. However, acceptance of a Calling within each person can serve as an antidote to devaluation. Could we accept the reality of millions of Helen Kellers?

While religions are held to the light of mirror in this paper, it is recognized that they have become strongly influenced in the recent century by scientific research and theories. Scientific findings and research techniques are taken for granted as reflections of reality, all too often, by non-scientists as secular scholarship is reified to provide direction and justification for social action. For example, it is often forgotten that the bell curve is simply a research tool, initially developed to compare and contrast samples within populations. It was designed to expand our understanding of our world; it has become a cage into which the entire world is distorted to forcibly fit. As such, it holds us back from seeing what is beyond its capacity to recognize and make sense of. For example: what if the reality of traits was not bell shaped, but spherical, as is taught within Native culture. Then, persons with outlier traits on one side of the sphere (I refrain from using the word, one end, there would be no end as reality would be nonlinear) could also have traits anywhere on other places in the sphere, such as at an opposite side. Thus, someone who is two standard deviations from the mean on one characteristic not appreciated within their culture, may also be two standard deviations from the mean on another characteristic that could be perceived within the culture as a significant contribution. (Or they may place anywhere else in the sphere as well.) It may help to envision a sphere such as the sun or earth as we proceed this imagining. There is a central core which is most dense, to correlate with the mean we see in the bell curve. As we move away from the central dense core into further layers, substance becomes less and less dense, to correlate with the more rare characteristics which occur as one moves from the center to the edges of the bell curve. However, to say that a cell occurs in the outer mantle does not disclose exactly where it occurs or whether it may move. How often have persons been identified as negative outliers on the bell curve who also retained incredibly rare artistic or other gifts that could have identified them also as a positive outlier, well beyond ordinary accomplishment! And how often is the mean, the dense core of ordinary experience, not normal at all, but simply a statistical identification of a mediocre average! Have we reified our tools to such a degree that we can not see beyond bell shapes?

Wolfensberger calls for us to create a "beloved community." Luckily, due to my ancestry, I found myself belonging within one. Most people are not so lucky. If they are to grow and become their potential it will be because we, as individuals, as educators, as religious leaders, as scientists have created such communities wherein devaluing is not ideologically rationalized and justified. I conclude with a proposal that we who return to the shared principle in Native American culture and western religion: that the life experience of each person can be a Divine Calling and that we do not use our religions, our sciences, our belief systems, our cultures as weapons of reductionistic authoritarianism that diminishes the quality and potential of any human life. "If we accept the concept of the life-creating, life-sustaining force or 'God' as omnipresent, it is not difficult to consider the next step. If God is omnipresent, God is in/with each and every one of us ... It may take a while for some of us to realize what our particular spiritual function is, but there most certainly is one. Above all–since we are each a part of God–each and every one of us is highly valuable. We must then treat each other–and ourselves–with respect and Love" (Samuels 1999, 86).

REFERENCES

Berger, P.L. and Luckman, T. (1967): *The Social Construction of Reality*. London: Allen Lane.

Bower, B. 2000: Raising Trust: Some Forager Groups May Nurture a Sharing Sense in Their Offspring. *Science News. Vol 158, No. 1, pp. 8-9.*

Conkin, P.K. (1968): *Puritans and Pragmatists*. Bloomington, IN.: Indiana University Press.

Curtis, N. (1987): *The Indians Book*. New York: Gramercy Books.

Davies, C.A. (1998): Constructing Other Selves: (In)competence and the Category of Learning Difficulties. Jenkins, R. *Questions of Competence: Culture, Classification and Intellectual Disability*. Cambridge: University Press.

Davis, R.D. & Braum, E.M. (1997): *The Gift of Dyslexia*. New York: Perigee.

Deland, J.S. (1999): Images of God Through the Lens of Disability. *Journal of Religion, Disability and Health. Vol. 3, No. 2, pp 47-81.*

Graymont, B. (1988): *The Iroquois*. New York: Chelsea Press.

Jenkins, R. (1998): *Questions of Competence: Culture, Classification and Intellectual Disability*. Cambridge: University Press.

Jenkins, R. (1998): Towards A Social Model of (In)competence. Jenkins, R. *Questions of Competence: Culture, Classification and Intellectual Disability.* Cambridge: University Press.

Joas, H. (1985): *G.H. Mead: A Contemporary Re-examination of his Thought.* Cambridge: M.I.T. Press.

Lundgren, N. (1999): Learning to Become (In)competent: Children in Belize. Jenkins, R. *Questions of Competence: Culture, Classification and Intellectual Disability.* Cambridge: University Press.

Nabokov, P. (Ed) (1991): *Native American Testimony.* New York: Penguin.

Nies, J. (1996): *Native American History.* New York: Ballantine Books.

Nuttall, M. (1999): States and Categories: Indigenous Models of Personhood in Northwest Greenland. Jenkins, R.: *Questions of Competence: Culture, Classification and Intellectual Disability.* Cambridge: University Press.

Oliver, M. (1990): *The Politics of Disability.* London: Macmillan.

Persons, S. (1983): *American Minds: A History of Ideas.* Malabar, FL: Robert E. Kreiger Publishers.

Reiter, S. (1999): Cross-Cultural Perspectives–Diversity and Universalism. Retish and Reiter: *Adults with Disabilities: International Perspectives in the Community.* Mahauh, NJ: Lawrence Erlbaum Assoc.

Retish, P. and Reiter, S. (Eds) (1999): *Adults with Disabilities: International Perspectives in the Community.* Mahwah, NJ: Lawrence Erlbaum Assoc.

Riley, P. (1993): *Growing Up Native American: An Anthrology.* New York: William Morrow.

Samuels, F. (1999): *To Spade the Earth.* New Durham, NH: Free Flow Press.

Schalock, R.L. and Kelly, C. (1999): Sociocultural Factors Influencing Social and Vocational Inclusion of Persons with Mental Retardation: A Cross-Cultural Study. Retish and Reiter: *Adults with Disabilities: International Perspectives in the Community.* Mahauh, NJ: Lawrence Erlbaum Assoc.

Szasz, T. (1969): The Myth of Mental Illness. Milton and Wahler (eds): *Behavior Disorders: Perspectives and Trends.* New York: J.B. Lippincott.

Taylor, C. (1989): *Sources of Self: The Making of the Modern Identity.* Cambridge: Harvard University Press.

Trent J.W. Jr. (1994): *Inventing the Feeble Mind: A History of Mental Retardation in the United States.* Berkeley: University of California Press.

Weber, M. (1976): *The Protestant Ethic and the Spirit of Capitalism.* New York: Charles Scribner.

Whyte, S.R. (1999): Slow Cookers and Madmen: Competence of Heart and Head in Rural Uganda. Jenkins, R.: *Questions of Competence: Culture, Classification, and Intellectual Disability.* Cambridge: University Press.

Wolfensberger, W. (1972): *The Principle of Normalization in Human Services.* Toronto: National Institute on Mental Retardation.

Open Wide the Doors to Christ: Persons with Intellectual Disabilities and the Roman Catholic Church

Kathy J. Smalley

SUMMARY. Persons with intellectual disabilities have always been included as members of the Roman Catholic Church. However, for centuries they were viewed as "holy innocents" who needed care but lacked the use of reason necessary for a mature faith life. In 1978, the National Conference of Catholic Bishops published a pastoral statement recognizing the needs and gifts of persons with disabilities. This pastoral and the two that followed have provided an impetus for "opening the doors" towards greater inclusion of persons with disabilities. This paper will explore the historical shifts in thinking and the present day relationship between persons with intellectual disabilities and the Church. Additionally, the spirituality of persons with intellectual disabilities will be highlighted. *[Article copies available for a fee from The Haworth Document Delivery Service: 1-800-342-9678. E-mail address: <getinfo@haworthpressinc.com> Website: <http://www.HaworthPress.com> © 2001 by The Haworth Press, Inc. All rights reserved.]*

KEYWORDS. Inclusion, Catholic, intellectual disabilities, spirituality, theology

---

Kathy J. Smalley was Director of the Office of Inclusion Ministry, Catholic Archdiocese of Seattle, Seattle WA, at the time this article was written.

[Haworth co-indexing entry note]: "Open Wide the Doors to Christ: Persons with Intellectual Disabilities and the Roman Catholic Church." Smalley, Kathy J. Co-published simultaneously in *Journal of Religion, Disability & Health* (The Haworth Pastoral Press, an imprint of The Haworth Press, Inc.) Vol. 5, No. 2/3, 2001, pp. 99-112; and: *Spirituality and Intellectual Disability: International Perspectives on the Effect of Culture and Religion on Healing Body, Mind, and Soul* (eds: William C. Gaventa, Jr. and David L. Coulter) The Haworth Pastoral Press, an imprint of The Haworth Press, Inc., 2001, pp. 99-112. Single or multiple copies of this article are available for a fee from The Haworth Document Delivery Service [1-800-342-9678, 9:00 a.m. - 5:00 p.m. (EST). E-mail address: getinfo@haworthpressinc.com].

Jesus said, *"I give praise to you, Father, Lord of heaven and earth for although you have hidden these things from the wise and the learned you have revealed them to the childlike" (Matthew 11: 25).*[1]

Persons with intellectual disabilities have always been included as members of the Roman Catholic Church. However, for centuries those labeled with such disabilities were viewed as less than whole human beings. Often considered "holy innocents," persons with intellectual disabilities were to be cared for and treated as "children of God," yet, they were denied reception of Sacraments and unable to participate fully in the faith life of the Church for they lacked the ability to reach the "age of reason."[2]

In 1978, the National Conference of Catholic Bishops of the United States (NCCB) published their first pastoral statement dedicated to persons with disabilities. Their emphasis and intent are reflected in the following remarks (NCCB, 1978):

> The same Jesus who heard the cry for recognition from the disabled of Judea and Samaria two thousand years ago calls us, his followers, to embrace our responsibility to our own disabled brothers and sisters in the United States. The Catholic Church pursues its mission by furthering the spiritual, intellectual, moral, and physical development of the people it serves. As pastors of the Church in America, we are committed to working for a deeper understanding of both the pain and the potential of our neighbors who are blind, deaf, mentally retarded, emotionally impaired, who have special learning problems, or who suffer from single or multiple physical disabilities—all those whom disability may set apart. We call upon people of good will to reexamine their attitudes toward their disabled brothers and sisters and promote their well-being, acting with the sense of justice and the compassion that the Lord so clearly desires. Further, realizing the unique gifts disabled individuals have to offer the Church, we wish to address the need for their fuller integration into the Christian community and their fuller participation in its life. (paragraph 1)

The *Pastoral Statement of U.S. Catholic Bishops on Persons with Disabilities* and the bishops' subsequent pastoral statements (i.e., *Guidelines for the Celebration of the Sacraments with Persons with Disabilities,* 1995; and *Welcome and Justice for Persons with Disabilities,* 1998) have provided an impetus for "opening the doors" towards greater inclusion of all persons with disabilities, including those with intellectual difficulties, in the total life of the Church.

This paper will briefly explore the historical shifts in society's thinking of and relating to persons with intellectual disabilities. The present day relationship between persons with intellectual disabilities and the Church will be highlighted. Additionally, the spirituality of persons with intellectual disabilities will be introduced through the use of anecdotes.

One of my greatest teachers has been a young woman named Lynn. She has severe epilepsy and intellectual disabilities. A few years ago during Lent, Lynn was quite taken by the Crucifixion. She couldn't understand why anyone would want to hurt Jesus. Again and again she asked very pointed and poignant questions about the how's and why's of the passion and death of Jesus. There was one question Lynn asked that I haven't forgot. In fact, this question is one that I frequently return to, turning it over and over in my mind. Still today, I am without an answer suitable for Lynn or myself.

Lynn, with hands on her hips and indignation in her voice, pointed at the Crucifix on the wall, and asked: "Kathy, when they killed Jesus and they hung him on that cross, where were his friends?"

(Where were his friends? Lynn, how do I answer you when I don't know the answer myself? Why did they abandon Jesus in his time of need? Why do we still abandon him today? You tell me, Lynn, for you are wiser than I am.)

HISTORY

Concerns of how to care for, live with, provide treatment or rehabilitation for, and interact with persons with intellectual disabilities have challenged society from the very beginning of time. Anthropological research has shown that human beings have an inherent need to classify objects (people, animals, characteristics, etc.). Classification allows humans to divide the objects into groups, which create structure and meaning. Grouping begins the process of separation that ultimately leads to acceptance for those who conform to the standard of measurement or exclusion and marginalization of those who don't. Categorizing or labeling persons as having intellectual disabilities almost certainly guarantees their marginalization.

Diane Bergant (1994) points out:

> People who do not fit into the classifications are frequently forced to live marginalized lives. When social institutions and structures are established according to patterns of normalcy, the inability of some people to conform prevents them from participating fully in the organizations or activities of the group. Too often they are regarded as less than human, their movement is restricted, their existence is circumscribed, and they are denied access to much that society offers for a fulfilling life. (p. 21)

Donald Senior (1998) equates a disabled person's marginalization with suffering:

> Being excluded is a form of suffering, one often more de-humanizing and more painful than physical disability itself. To be excluded from participating in a group or function diminishes a person. Exclusion implies that someone is less than human, not capable or worthy of participating in normal human discourse. It is a form of suffering that disabled persons in particular are made to bear. (p. 7)

Jean Vanier (1998, p. 72), the founder of the international federation of communities known as L'Arche, says, "I have come to the conclusion that those with intellectual disabilities are among the most oppressed and excluded people in the world." While Vanier was speaking of the present day relationship between society and persons with intellectual disabilities, his statement would hold true throughout most of history.

Before Jesus' birth, persons with intellectual disabilities were killed by the Spartan Greek society. Alternatively, in Roman society, people with mental retardation were used as forms of entertainment (fools or jesters) for the leadership and the wealthy (Webb-Mitchell, 1994, p. 52).

Parts of early Judaic law regarded persons with disabilities as unclean and unworthy as evidenced in this except from the book of Leviticus:

> The Lord said to Moses, "Speak to Aaron and tell him: None of your descendants, of whatever generation, who has any defect, shall come forward to offer the food of his God. Therefore, he who has any of the following defects may not come forward: he who is

blind, or lame, or who has any disfigurement or malformation, or a crippled foot or hand, or who is humpbacked or weakly or walleyed, or who is afflicted with eczema, ringworm or hernia. No descendant of Aaron the priest who has any such defect may draw near to offer up the oblations of the Lord; on account of his defect he may not draw near to offer up the food of his God." (Leviticus 21: 16-22)

The beginning of Jesus' public ministry brought significant transformation to "life as usual" in Judea. Jesus said, "Do not think that I have come to bring peace upon the earth. I have come to bring not peace but the sword" (Matthew 10:34). He proclaimed he was the Son of God, challenged the people to love one another, and spoke of the coming of the Kingdom.

Additionally, Jesus showed the people a different way to treat persons with intellectual disabilities and all persons who are marginalized:

At that time the disciples approached Jesus and said, "Who is the greatest in the kingdom of heaven?" He called a child over, placed the child in their midst, and said, "Amen, I say to you, unless you turn and become like children, you will not enter the kingdom of heaven. Whoever humbles himself like this child is the greatest in the kingdom of heaven. And whoever receives one child such as this in my name receives me." (Matthew 18:1-5)

In fact, Jesus purposely sought out those considered unclean and unholy: people with leprosy (Mark 1:40-45; Luke 17:11-19), people thought to be possessed by demons (Matthew 17:14-21; Mark 1:21-28; 5:1-20), and people with sensory impairments (Mark 7:31-37; 10:46-52). (Reid, 1994, p. 44)

Throughout the New Testament one can find reference to Jesus fulfilling the words of the prophets. In the Gospel of Matthew (8:16-17) it is said:

When it was evening, they brought him many who were possessed by demons, and he drove out the spirits by a word and cured all the sick, to fulfill what had been said by Isaiah the prophet: He took away our infirmities and bore our diseases.

Barbara Reid (p. 45) explains the significance of Jesus' fulfillment of this particular passage in Matthew; "The most radical step of all is not simply that Jesus associates with those considered unclean, but that Jesus himself assumes such an identity. In doing so, Jesus redefines the notions of 'holy' and 'unholy.' "

One could argue that Jesus hanging on the cross at the time of his Crucifixion had taken on the persona of a man with multiple disabling conditions. Jesus' vulnerability links him with all those who are helpless and vulnerable. God's plan called for Jesus to both come into the world and leave the world as one who was totally helpless. Paul Wadell (1994) explains why it is necessary to understand Jesus' helplessness:

> Seeing Jesus as the norm of all things human reverses our sense of being human. Our neediness is not something about which to be ashamed, but the door through which God's love enters our lives. Our dependence is not a weakness, but a prerequisite for fullness of life; indeed, the truth of our nature is our absolute need to receive. To the extent we are able to acknowledge our need, we receive life which blesses us far more than we ever could ourselves. To be ashamed of our need is thus to be needlessly deprived. (p. 62)

Early Christians, after the death and resurrection of Jesus, tried to live a communal life where everyone's needs were met. The goal was to create "the Body of Christ"[3] in their midst. Thus, persons with intellectual disabilities were to be cared for by the community. However, as time went by and the community of Christians continued to grow, the Church became unable to meet the needs of all its members.

Using people with intellectual disabilities as jesters for the amusement of others did not occur only in the Roman era. In the early Middle Ages of Europe, such practices were commonplace. As Brett Webb-Mitchell recounts, even Pope Leo X (1513-1521) had such entertainers at his dinners:

> Buffoons and jesters [who] were nearly always to be found at his table where the guests were encouraged to laugh at their antics and at the cruel jokes which were played on them—as when, for instance, some half-witted, hungry dwarf was seen guzzling a plate of carrion covered in a strong sauce under the impression that he was being privileged to consume the finest fare. (p. 60)

The early Middle Ages also saw the beginning of hospices and hospitals for the ill and the "feeble-minded." Most of these sanctuaries where developed by monastic orders of men or women and provided persons with intellectual disabilities compassionate care and a sense of safety.

Unfortunately over time, some of these facilities became houses of terror and torture instead of havens of comfort and care.

The 15th and 16th centuries brought much turbulence to society. A combination of the plague, famine due to crop failures, and increasing corruption in the church and in society created intense needs for shelter, food, healthcare, etc. The Church was overwhelmed with demands for assistance and subsequently those with disabilities received little or no help.

During this tumultuous time new ideas were taking hold and the Protestant Reformation occurred. Both Catholic and Protestant theology emphasized the belief in a vengeful God. The need for personal redemption as well as personal responsibility permeated society. Thus, those who could not take responsibility for themselves (e.g., persons with intellectual disabilities) were not worthy and often were persecuted. One example of such treatment is the Salem witch trials.

As the United States grew, religious orders from Europe sent their sisters, brothers, and priests to work with the immigrant settlers. Soon hospitals and homes for the disabled were established in this country. Often these homes grew into large institutions designed to keep the residents separate from society. People with disabilities were still considered shameful secrets who were to be "kept in the closet."

It wasn't until after World War I and World War II when fathers and brothers, uncles and cousins were coming home with missing limbs, sensory impairments, and emotional illnesses, that persons with disabilities became visible in society.

I had the opportunity to fill in as a temporary chaplain at Northern Center, a state institution for persons with developmental disabilities. Each week, as part of my duties, I would lead two communion services.

On my first day at Northern Center I met a young man named Steve. He was a tall, handsome, blond man and except for the jagged scar, which ran across his forehead, he looked "normal." Steve had been in a car accident around the age of 9 or 10 and had suffered significant brain damage, including impulse control.

Steve liked to come to the Wednesday evening communion service so he could help the staff bring the residents in wheelchairs down to the conference room we used for the service. He also liked to ask questions and share his experiences and insights into God and Church and faith.

One wintry Wednesday evening I was running late. I also was less than cheerful having spent the last few hours negotiating the snowy roads. When I arrived Steve was already waiting for me.

He started in with his usual barrage of questions and I told him, rather sharply, that I was too busy to talk. Steve was undisturbed by my harsh tones and kept up his banter. He picked up the crucifix I had set on the table and said, "You know, Kathy, this is Jesus." I'm sure I nodded and said something like, "You're right, Steve." Then Steve picked up the ciborium[4] and removed its lid. He pointed at the consecrated hosts and said, "And this is Jesus, too." I was impressed that he could make the connection but the room was beginning to fill and I shooed him away to help with the other residents (and more importantly to leave me alone).

Well, it was one of those nights. Every time I would say something Steve would butt in with a story or a question. "Kathy, if Mary is Jesus' mother who is God's mother?" "Kathy, you want to know what angels are? They're little holy ghosts." "Kathy, why didn't God come down to be Jesus' father instead of Joseph?" And so on. I was slowly losing what little patience I had left.

Finally, it was time for Communion. Because most of the residents were non-ambulatory I would go to them to distribute Communion. Steve always wanted to be first. I placed the host in his hands and turned towards the next resident. From over my shoulder I heard Steve say, "Kathy, this is Jesus." "Yes, Steve, I know," I snapped, "Now put the host in your mouth."

"No, Kathy. Look. Jesus is on here," he said very intently as he looked into his hands. I knew that if I didn't go back and look, he wouldn't stop bugging me. So I looked at the host in Steve's hands. On that host was a stamped crucifix and the corpus of Jesus. "I see Steve," I said, "You're right it is Jesus. Now please put the host in your mouth."

I finished distributing Communion and on the way back to the front of the room I looked at the half-dozen or so hosts left in the ciborium. None of them had anything stamped on them. After the service was finished, I took the ciborium back to the church in town. I knew where Father kept a bag of unconsecrated hosts and out of curiosity I looked for one like the one I had seen in Steve's hands. There were none.

Each week for the six months that I was chaplain I looked for a host with a stamped crucifix and corpus. I never found one.

PRESENT DAY

The 1960s brought a concerted effort towards meeting the needs of persons with disabilities. The first strong federal legislation designed to provide education, employment, and housing for persons with disabilities was enacted. The Kennedy family spearheaded services and treatment for persons with intellectual disabilities. Additionally, they established the Special Olympics program (Krafft, 1988, p. 19).

The 1960s also saw the beginning of community-based residential housing and the start of the "de-institutionalization" of the state-run institutions. This trend helped bring persons with disabilities back into their communities, stores, schools, places of worship, and the like.

A third significant change for persons with intellectual disabilities, which involved the Catholic Church, also took place during the 1960s. The National Apostolate for the Mentally Retarded (NAMR) was established in 1968. NAMR's original mission was to work for the total integration of the mentally retarded in the life of the Church and the life of the community and their first Episcopal Advisor was Cardinal Cushing. Much of NAMR's early work was in the area of religious education for persons with intellectual disabilities (Pesaniello, 1998, pages 5-6).

According to Browne (1997, pages 51-52), "The waters of change washing through so many areas of our society had at long last reached the disabled, acknowledging them as a specifically identifiable group with definable concerns within the social awareness of the Church."

The Pastoral Statement of U.S. Catholic Bishops on Persons with Disabilities was published on November 16, 1978. Early in the pastoral the bishops acknowledge the past shortcomings of the Church:

> The Church, through the response of its members to the needs of their neighbors, and through its parishes, health care institutions, and social service agencies, has always attempted to show a pastoral concern for disabled individuals. However, in a spirit of humble candor, we must acknowledge that at times we have responded to the needs of some of our disabled people only after circumstances or public opinion have compelled us to do so. (paragraph 6)

The bishops go on to outline their vision for persons with disabilities and the ecclesial community. They emphasize the need of inclusion at the local, diocesan, and national levels. The bishops say:

> For most Catholics, the community of believers is embodied in the local parish. The parish is the door to participation for persons with disabilities, and it is the responsibility of the pastor and lay leaders to make sure that this door is always open. (paragraph 17)

Additionally, the bishops tell their pastors:

> It is essential that all forms of the liturgy be completely accessible
> to persons with disabilities, since these forms are the essence of
> the spiritual tie that binds the Christian community together. To
> exclude members of the parish from these celebrations of the life
> of the Church, even by passive omission, is to deny the reality of
> that community. (paragraph 22)

In 1995, the NCCB published their second pastoral statement on disabilities: *Guidelines for the Celebration of the Sacraments with Persons with Disabilities*. Here the bishops wrote:

> These guidelines were developed to address many of the concerns
> raised by priests, pastoral ministers, other concerned Catholics,
> persons with disabilities, their advocates and their families of
> greater consistency in pastoral practice in the celebration of the
> sacraments throughout the country. With this objective in view,
> the guidelines draw upon the Church's ritual books, its canonical
> tradition, and its experience in ministering to or with persons with
> disabilities in order to dispel any misunderstandings that may im-
> pede sound pastoral practice in the celebration of the sacraments.
> (p. 2)

The guidelines document begins with seven general principles,
which can be summarized as follows:

1. By reason of their baptism, all Catholics are equal in dignity in the
   sight of God, and have the same calling.
2. Catholics with disabilities have a right to participate in the sacraments as full functioning members of the local ecclesial community.
3. Parish sacramental celebrations should be accessible to persons
   with disabilities and open to their full, active and conscious participation, according to their capacity.
4. Since the parish is the center of the Christian experience for most
   Catholics, pastoral ministers should make every effort to determine the presence of all Catholics with disabilities who reside
   within a parish's boundaries.
5. Pastors are responsible to be as inclusive as possible in providing
   evangelization, catechetical formation, and sacramental preparation for parishioners with disabilities.

6. The creation of a fully accessible parish reaches beyond mere physical accommodation to encompass the attitudes of all parishioners towards persons with disabilities.
7. Dioceses are encouraged to establish appropriate policies for handling [difficult] cases which respect the procedural and substantive rights of all involved, and which ensure the necessary provision of consultation. (pp. 2-5)

Following the general principles, the bishops address each of the seven sacraments[5] individually. It is within the discussion for the sacraments of Confirmation, Eucharist, and Penance that the bishops address persons with intellectual disabilities who can never reach the age of reason:

> Persons who because of developmental or mental disabilities may never attain the use of reason are to be encouraged either directly or, if necessary, through their parents or guardian, to receive the sacrament of confirmation at the appropriate time. (p.8)

On the twentieth anniversary (1998) of their first pastoral statement, the NCCB released *Welcome and Justice for Persons with Disabilities: A Framework of Access and Inclusion.* It is a reaffirmation of ten of the principles from their two earlier statements. They say:

> This moral framework is based upon Catholic documents and serves as a guide for contemplation and action. We hope that the reaffirmation of the following principles will assist the faithful in bringing the principles of justice and inclusion to the many new and evolving challenges confronted by persons with disabilities today. (paragraph 2)

The bishops use this latest document to reaffirm the uniqueness of each human being and acknowledge the dignity of persons with disabilities. They also condemn the culture of death, which seeks to destroy through abortion, physician-assisted suicide, and medical rationing while defending the right to life for all human beings, including those with intellectual disabilities (no. 1-4).

The Catholic Church in the United States has begun to recognize persons with intellectual disabilities as more than poor souls who only need our care and our prayers due, in part, to the NCCB's documents. Today, parishes throughout the country and in other parts of the world, as well, are inviting persons with intellectual disabilities to worship together, to use their unique gifts in service to the parish, and to be included as full participating members of the Church's community.

The Church's movement towards full inclusion for persons with intellectual disabilities is based on the practices and words of Jesus and it seeks to affirm what Jean Vanier has said:

> The point of inclusion is the belief that each of us is important, unique, sacred, in fact. We can only relate to others and begin to include them in our lives and our society if we have this primary belief. Our basic needs are the same as those of all other human beings. We need other people who will call forth what is most beautiful in us, just as we need to call forth what is most beautiful in others. (p. 95)

The prophetic words of the U.S. Catholic bishops (1978) guarantee commitment toward and vigilance for opening wide the doors to Christ to persons with intellectual disabilities:

> No one would deny that every man, woman, and child has the right to develop his or her potential to the fullest. With God's help and our own determination, the day will come when that right is realized in the lives of all persons with disabilities (paragraph 33). Persons with disabilities are not looking for pity. They seek to serve the community and to enjoy their full baptismal rights as members of the Church. Our interaction with them can and should be an affirmation of our faith. There can be no separate Church for persons with disabilities. We are one flock that follows a single shepherd. (paragraph 32)

I was asked by the group home manager to meet with John. John was a man in his late 30s or early 40s with intellectual disabilities and some challenging behavioral problems. Unfortunately, John had become loud and agitated during Mass at his life-long parish. After the Mass, the pastor told John that he could no longer come to the church. John became upset and began hurling four-letter suggestions at the pastor. This did not help the situation, as one might imagine. Consequently, the pastor made it clear to John and the staff at the group home that he was not welcome and the police would be called if he tried to come onto parish property.

During one of our early visits I asked John how he felt about being banned from the church he had grown up in. I will never forget John's answer. He said, "Kathy, at first I was angry with the people and the priest for being afraid of me and telling me I couldn't come anymore. But, then I realized that God is like a jigsaw puzzle."

Since I didn't see the connection I asked him to explain.

He said, "Each of us is a person and we all are different from other people. And each of us experiences who God is but because we are different from other people our ideas about God are different, too. And God is even bigger than anyone's ideas. And a jigsaw puzzle is made up of little pieces. All the pieces are different just like people. And you can't see what the picture is until you put all the different pieces together. So, in a way, it's like God is this huge jigsaw puzzle made up of each of our different pieces. And we can't see the face of God until we put the puzzle together."

Then John's face broke into a huge grin and he said, "Kathy, guess what? I've got the last piece to the puzzle and they can't see God without me!"

NOTES

1. All biblical references are taken from *The New American Bible, Saint Joseph Edition (1970)*. New York, NY: Catholic Book Publishing Company.

2. The age of reason is defined as the time of life at which a person is assumed to be morally responsible and able to distinguish between right and wrong. It is generally held to be by the end of the seventh year.

3. The phrase "Body of Christ" is part of Pauline theology. It first appears in Romans chapter 12 ("For as in one body we have many parts, and all the parts do not have the same function, so we, though many, are one body in Christ." verses 4-5). Other references include 1st Corinthians chapter 12 and Ephesians chapter 4.

4. A ciborium is defined as a covered container used to hold consecrated small hosts. It is similar to a chalice but covered and larger and is made of various precious metals, and the interior is commonly gold or gold-plated.

5. A sacrament is defined as a sensible sign, instituted by Jesus Christ, by which invisible grace and inward sanctification are communicated to the soul. In the Roman Catholic Church there are seven sacraments: Baptism, Eucharist, Penance, Confirmation, Matrimony, Holy Orders, and the Sacrament of the Sick.

REFERENCES

Bergant, Dianne, C.S.A. (1994). "Come, let us go up to the mountain of the Lord" (Isa 2:3): Biblical Reflections on the Question of Sacramental Access. In Edward Foley (Ed.), *Developmental Disabilities and Sacramental Access* (pp. 13-32). Collegeville, MN: The Liturgical Press.

Browne, Elizabeth J., Ph.D. (1997). *The Disabled Disciple: Ministering in a Church Without Barriers*. Liguori, MO: Liguori Publications.

Krafft, Jane, M.S.B.T. (1988). *The Ministry to Persons with Disabilities*. Collegeville, MN: The Liturgical Press.

Pesaniello, Matthew, M. Rev. (1998, Summer). Why A "National Apostolate for the Mentally Retarded?" *National Apostolate for Inclusion Ministry*, 5-6.

Reid, Barbara, O.P. (1994). The Whole Broken Body of Christ–New Testament Reflections on Access to the Holy through Jesus. In Edward Foley (Ed.), *Developmental Disabilities and Sacramental Access*. (pp. 33-52). Collegeville, MN: The Liturgical Press.

Senior, Donald, C.P. (1998). Suffering as Inaccessibility: Lessons from the New Testament Healing Stories. *New Theology Review*, *l* (4), 5-14.

United States Catholic Conference. (1978). *Pastoral Statement of U.S. Catholic Bishops on Persons with Disabilities*. [Brochure]. National Conference of Catholic Bishops.

United States Catholic Conference. (1995). *Guidelines for the Celebration of the Sacraments with Persons with Disabilities*. [Brochure]. National Conference of Catholic Bishops.

United States Catholic Conference. (1998). *Welcome and Justice for Persons with Disabilities*. [Brochure]. National Conference of Catholic Bishops.

Vanier, Jean. (1998). *Becoming Human*. Mahwah, NJ: Paulist Press.

Wadell, Paul J., C.P. (1994). Pondering the Anomaly of God's Love. In Edward Foley (Ed.), *Developmental Disabilities and Sacramental Access* (pp. 53-72). Collegeville, MN: The Liturgical Press.

Webb-Mitchell, Brett. (1994). *Unexpected Guests at God's Banquet: Welcoming People with Disabilities Into the Church*. New York: The Crossroads Publishing Company.

III. BRINGING SCIENCE INTO SPIRITUALITY: RESEARCH AND PRACTICE

Spiritual Health and Persons with Intellectual Disability: A Review

Joav Merrick, MD, DMSc
Mohammed Morad, MD
Udi Levy, MA

SUMMARY. Religion and faith seems to play an important part in medicine and health in spite of the advances of modern medicine. This presentation reviews the present knowledge of the interaction between prayer, religious activity, distant healing and health in general and the few studies involving religion and persons with intellectal disability. Re-

Joav Merrick is the Medical Director of the Division for Mental Retardation in Israel, Ministry of Labour and Social Affairs, P.O. Box 1260, IL-91012 Jerusalem, Israel (E-mail: jmerrick@aquanet.co.il). Mohammed Morad is Family Physician at the Department of Family Medicine at Ben Gurion University, Beer Sheva, Israel. Udi Levy is the Director of Kfar Rafael, Beer Sheva, Israel, a unique residential care center for persons with intellectual disability living in a kibbutz-like facility of seven families caring for nearly 50 persons with intellectual disability.

[Haworth co-indexing entry note]: "Spiritual Health and Persons with Intellectual Disability: A Review." Merrick, Joav, Mohammed Morad, and Udi Levy. Co-published simultaneously in *Journal of Religion, Disability & Health* (The Haworth Pastoral Press, an imprint of The Haworth Press, Inc.) Vol. 5, No. 2/3, 2001, pp. 113-121; and: *Spirituality and Intellectual Disability: International Perspectives on the Effect of Culture and Religion on Healing Body, Mind, and Soul* (eds: William C. Gaventa, Jr. and David L. Coulter) The Haworth Pastoral Press, an imprint of The Haworth Press, Inc., 2001, pp. 113-121. Single or multiple copies of this article are available for a fee from The Haworth Document Delivery Service [1-800-342-9678, 9:00 a.m. - 5:00 p.m. (EST). E-mail address: getinfo@haworthpressinc.com].

113

sults from a recent study of spiritual health in residential centers for persons with intellectual disability are also reviewed. It is concluded that there indeed seems to be a connection between spiritual activities and physical health and well-being. *[Article copies available for a fee from The Haworth Document Delivery Service: 1-800-342-9678. E-mail address: <getinfo@haworthpressinc.com> Website: <http://www.HaworthPress.com>* © *2001 by The Haworth Press, Inc. All rights reserved.]*

KEYWORDS. Intellectual disability, spiritual health, spiritual activity, residential care, Israel

In 1882 the philosopher Friedrich Nietzsche proclaimed that G-d was dead (Armstrong 1999), but inspite of Nietzsche, the 20th century with the two World Wars and the fall of the Russian Empire, people around this world still believe in G-d.

Religion and faith seem to play a part in medicine and health also. A study from the Evans County Cardiovascular Epidemiological Study 1967-69 (Graham et al., 1978) showed a consistant pattern of lower systolic and diastolic blood pressures among frequent church attenders compared to that of infrequent attenders, which was not due to the effects of age, obesity, smoking or socioeconomic status. At the San Francisco General Medical Center a prospective randomized double-blind study was conducted over ten months with 393 patients admitted to the Coronary Care Unit (Byrd, 1988) with 192 patients assigned to an intercessory prayer group and 201 patients as control group. The prayer group had significantly lower severity score based on the hospital course after entry, the control group required more frequent ventilatory assistance, antibiotics and diuretics and it seemed that prayer had a beneficial therapeutic effect on coronary disease.

The Dartmouth Medical School in New Hampshire looked at risk prevention in 232 patients within six months of cardiac surgery (Oxman et al., 1995) and found that three biomedical variables were significant predictors of mortality: history of previous cardiac surgery, greater impairment in presurgery basic activities of daily living and older age. Among the social and religious risk factors were lack of participation in social and community groups and absence of strength and comfort from religion.

The Duke University Medical Center in North Carolina examined (Koenig et al., 1998) the relationship between religious activities and blood pressure in 3,963 community dwelling adults aged 65 years and older. The religiously active tended to have lower blood pressures than those less active and the findings applied to attendance at religious services and private religious activities, but not to religious media (religious television watching or listening radio programs).

The Geraldine Brush Cancer Research Institute in San Francisco (Sicher et al., 1998) in a double-blind randomized trial studied 40 patients with advanced AIDS (Acquired Immunodeficiency Syndrome) and the effects of distant healing with prayer and psychic healing. The healers were located throughout the United States during the study and the subjects and healers never met. After six months of distant healing the treatment subjects showed significantly fewer new AIDS-defining illnesses, had lower illness severity, required significantly fewer physician visits, fewer hospitalizations and fewer days of hospitalizations. The treated subjects also showed improved mood compared to controls.

A recent study from the Coronary Care Unit at the Mid America Heart Institute in Kansas City (Harris et al., 1999) replicated the study by Byrd (1988) and also found that supplementary, remote, blinded, intercessory prayer produced a measurable improvement in the medical outcomes of critically ill patients.

STUDIES ON SPIRITUAL HEALTH AND PERSONS WITH INTELLECTUAL DISABILITY

There are only a few studies on religion, religious services or activities, prayer and health in the population of persons with disability and especially intellectual disability (ID). The Institute for Health, Health Care Policy and Aging Research at Rutgers University (Idler & Kasl, 1997) has looked at health practices, social activities, well-being and attendance or religious services as a predictor of the course of disability in a population of non-institutionalized community dwelling elderly persons (2,812 persons with an average age of 74.5 years) from New Haven, who were interviewed annually from 1982 through 1989. Disability (like stroke, diabetes, broken bones, amputation, etc.) was composed of 15 items and rated from "some difficulty" to "unable to do." The studies showed that religious involvement was tied to a broad array of behavioral and psychosocial resources, that these resources were associated with attendance at services and some of these associations were especially pronounced among disabled elderly persons. Their longitudinal study with a 12 years follow-up showed that attendance at services was a strong predictor of better functioning, that health practices, social ties and indicators of well-being reduced, but did not eliminate these effects, and that disability had minimal effects on subsequent attendance. The studies showed that religious participation had an impact on health and well-being of elderly people and especially these with an disability.

One study of 102 families having a 3-5 year old child (Weisner et al., 1991) from the Los Angeles metropolitan area with developmental delay of uncertain etiology showed that religious parents described the purpose of their children with delays in their lives in emotionally powerful and meaningful ways that clearly helped them, even though direct measures of peace of mind and emotional adjustment did not differ with non-religious families. Religion seemed to play a powerful role for the families in explaining misfortune and suffering more than a practical way to provide support or organizing specific beliefs and accommodations. The families were Christian or Jewish and none were practising Hindus, Muslims or Buddhists.

Another study of 52 African-American caregivers, living in a southern California urban community, and having a child with intellectual disability (Rogers-Dulan, 1998) showed that religion in personal and family life and church support had a positive effect on adjustment for these families. These positive effect outcomes were focused on the need for assistance and help in the face of challenge and struggle, meaning and a moral or ethical path to good and a source of hope and peace. Most of the responses by the families to these themes were positive, but there were three categories of negative statements: some members of organized religious groups did not assist or were not helpful to them, they avoided organized religion and they expressed feelings of guilt and thought that they were being punished by God. All participants, though, did express a belief in a personal God.

OUR EXPERIENCES FROM A STUDY IN ISRAEL

Today in Israel there is a total population of 6,037,000 persons, and the Division for Mental Retardation (DMR) under the Ministry of Labour and Social Affairs is in contact with close to 20,000 persons (all ages). Residential care is provided to about 6,022 persons in 53 institutions or residential centers (Merrick, 1999) all over the country. Another 1,700 persons are provided residential care in hostels or protected apartments in communities in about another 50 places; the other 12,300 persons are served with day-care kindergarten, day-treatment centers, sheltered workshops or integrated care in the community.

The 6,022 persons with ID in residential care are located in nine government, 32 private and 12 public residential centers with a mean of 113.62 persons in each institution (range 22-398). The population of these 53 residential centers was the focus of a recent study of spiritual health activities (Merrick et al., 2000)

In this study a questionnaire was constructed with free-answer questions with the following contents:

1. The concept of spiritual health.
2. The difference between spiritual and emotional.
3. Spiritual activity in the residential center.
4. Spiritual activity on an individual scale and on a communal scale at the residential center.
5. Activity through the staff and activity upon request.
6. Expression of spiritual activity on an individual level.
7. The family involvement in spiritual activity.
8. The attitude of the staff towards the contribution of spiritual activity to the health and well-being of the residents.
9. Suggestions by staff towards enriching the spiritual world of the residents.
10. Readiness by staff to cooperate in future activities to enhance the spiritual life of the residents.

The questionnaire was mailed to all directors of 53 residential centers in Israel caring for persons with ID resulting in the return of 25 questionnaires (response rate of 47%). The responders were directors, psychologists, social workers, education officers or medical personnel. In 50% of responses the participants defined spiritual health as the inner world of a person in balance with a healthy feeling, and 60% defined this as a process accompanied by positive feelings like happiness, calm, relaxation, quietness and contentment, during internal and interpersonal communication.

Five of the responders expressed explicit difficulties with the concept of spiritual health. A large proportion of the responders (33%) related complete importance to the presence of intellect as a condition for experience of spiritual health.

Nearly half of the responders (45%) expressed an undeniable relationship between the physical, mental and spiritual body and the importance of harmony among them. Some defined this as a feeling of the person's belonging to general concepts like God (15%), and some related it to the universal spiritual realm that exists in every person (1/25). Three responders (12%) stated the importance of spiritual health as a give and take situation between the person and his surroundings.

Three related to spiritual health as a therapeutic affect in times of pressure and distress that command the body and mind (12%). The connection between spiritual health and worship, prayer, holidays and religious rituals was only mentioned in 12% of the responses.

The majority of the responders stated that spiritual health was a subjective feeling connected to the person's grasp of his world based upon a balance built by religious, philosophical and social standards like culture and the arts, whereas mental health was looked upon as an objective state. A small number of responders (5/25) expressed difficulty in separating the two forms of health.

In relation to mental health, most of the responders defined it as *different,* because of their understanding that it is tied more to the body and physical ability of the person as opposed to the spiritual, which a portion of the responders believed is more free from the body.

The activities perceived as spiritual by the staff of the residential centers were varied (examples include: theater, song, yoga, sport, meditation, zoo-therapy, music therapy, imagination workshops, therapeutic conversations, religious holidays, etc.), but were mainly managed in groups and existed in only some of the centers (average of activity per center was 3.56). For the majority (23/25), the staff members were the ones, who planned and ran the activities. The staff did not incorporate spiritual activity and guidance at an individual level and according to the responses, there did not seem to be awareness of such activity.

Most of the spiritual activity reported in most of the residential centers was in the religious area, including: holidays, upholding the commandments, making kiddush (sanctification of the Sabbath), separation of the sexes and modest dress.

The character of the activities in the residential centers matched the concept of spiritual health. Therefore, whenever there was a religious concept it was expressed in the answers, with a main focus on religion. A portion of the residential centers (3/25) gave no report of spiritual activity. From about half of the responses it became clear that the parents were involved and were encouraging spiritual activity not only on an individual level, but also in the communal level within the residential center and with the community outside of it. In nine centers (36%) there was no parental involvement in this activity and in two places no answer was given at all regarding parental involvement of this kind.

In 96% (24/25) of the residential centers, the responders believed and were convinced that there is a clear and decisive contribution to the spiritual health of the residents through the activities performed. The survey also revealed that 84% (21/25) of the participants expressed their readiness to be involved in discussions or activities to prepare, plan and enrich the spiritual life of the person with intellectual disability.

DISCUSSION

The importance of clergy, churches, synagogues, mosques, other houses of worship and faith communities is often not recognized in the work with families with children with intellectual disability, even though many families have a need for continuous support from their clergy or congregation, when their support system breaks down (Heifetz, 1987). In spite of attempts at "matchmaking" between the worlds of religious and secular services (Heifetz, 1987), there is still a long way to go.

There are several studies on service personnel (such as: physicians, nurses, and residential care staff) regarding their religious beliefs and their attitudes towards religion and healing. One survey from the United States (Koenig et al., 1991) on religious denomination, showed that belief in a higher power, church attendance, and religious coping (among the 130 physicians, 39 nurses, 77 patients and 60 family members) revealed that a large proportion of patients and families looked upon religion as an important factor–a factor which enabled them to cope; whereas only a small percentage of physicians felt that way.

Physicians from Holland (Kuyck et al., 2000) responded to a postal questionnaire (120 general practitioners (GP) with 87 responses). When a patient registered in their practice 16% of the GPs paid attention to the religious beliefs of the patient, whereas 79% of the GPs paid attention, only when it was a case of end-of-life decisions. A GP with a Protestant background tended to pay more attention to religious beliefs in this study than physicians with a Catholic background (65% versus 36%).

From Canada there is one report (Porter, 1998) of pastoral support for a Jewish adult with developmental disabilities in a predominantly Christian setting. This case report outlines the growth in self-esteem in the adult and the resulting transformation into interfaith awareness and appreciation of the author in the surrounding Jewish and Christian communities.

Our study (Merrick et al., 2000) showed that spiritual activity was a part of the programs for persons with intellectual disability in residential care in Israel, but the activities were varied and lacked a planned or uniform character. This is surely due to many factors, but could be due, in part, to: the subjective definition of what spiritual health entails, the individual perception of activities, and, maybe, the lack of scientific proof that spiritual health activities improve the health of persons with intellectual disability.

Due to the diversity of definitions of spiritual health and, the interesting observation from our study, that nearly any activity was defined as spiritual would make it very difficult to find a universal platform for providing spiritual health promotion for the population of persons with intellectual disability in residential care. There is no formal policy on the level of the Ministry of Labour and Social Affairs in the field of spiritual health and, therefore, the activities taking place are largely dependent on the philosophical, secular or religious beliefs or affiliations of the administrators and the staff at the residential centers.

Parental involvement was observed to a great extent in our study and this interest, together with the positive attitude of the care staff, should make the challenge to increase spiritual health activities a priority in this population in the future.

CONCLUSION

Spiritual health as a phenomena was reviewed and several studies showed a connection between spiritual activity, spiritual health and physical health improvements. One study, conducted in a population of persons with intellectual disability through a questionnaire method, found variations in the care staff's perception of the definition of spiritual health, and variations in the activities at the residential centers categorized as spiritual activity, but revealed a clear and positive parental involvement.

It is believed a great challenge to try to carry out an intervention activity program in this population, and the earlier 1987 call for match-making (Heifetz, 1987) between secular and religious efforts can only be repeated.

REFERENCES

Armstrong, K. (1999). Where has God gone? *Newsweek*, July 12, 54-55.
Byrd, R.C. (1988). Positive therapeutic effects of intercessory prayer in a coronary care unit population. *South Medical Journal* 81(7), 826-829.
Graham, T.W., Kaplan, B.H., Cornoni-Huntley, J.C., James, S.A., Becker, C., Hames, C.G. & Heyden, S. (1978). Frequency of church attendance and blood pressure elevation. *Journal of Behavioral Medicine* 1(1), 37-43.

Harris, W.S., Gowda, M., Kolb, J.W., Strychacz, C.P., Vacek, J.L., Jones, P.G., Forker, A., O'Keefe, J.H. & McCallister B.D. (1999). A randomized, controlled trial of the effects of remote, intercessory prayer on outcomes in patients admitted to the coronary care unit. *Archives of Internal Medicine*, 159(19), 2273-2278.

Heifetz, L.J. (1987). Integrating religious and secular perspectives in the design and delivery of disability services. *Mental Retardation*, 25, 127-131.

Idler, E.L. & Kasl, S.V. (1997). Religion among disabled and nondisabled persons I: Cross-sectional patterns in health practices, social activities and well-being. *Journal of Gerontology: Social Sciences*, 52B(6), S294-305.

Idler, E.L. & Kasl, S.V. (1997). Religion among disabled and nondisabled persons II: Attendance ar religious services as a predictor of the course of disability. *Journal of Gerontology: Social Sciences*, 52B(6), S306-316.

Koenig, H.G., Bearon, L.B., Hover, M & Travis, J.L. (1991). Religious perspectives of doctors, nurses, patients and families. *Journal of Pastoral Care* 45(3), 254-267.

Koenig, H.G., George, L.K., Hays, J.C., Larson, D.B., Cohen, H.J. & Blazer, D.G. (1998). The relationship between religious activities and blood pressure in older adults. *International Journal of Psychiatry and Medicine*, 28(2), 189-213.

Kuyck, W.G. (2000). Do doctors pay attention to the religious beliefs of their patients ? A survey among Dutch GPs. *Family Practice* 17(3), 230-232.

Merrick, J. (1999). Survey of medical clinics serving persons with intellectual disability in residential care in Israel 1998. Jerusalem, Israel: Ministry of Labour and Social Affairs, 1999.

Merrick, J., Morad, M. & Levy, U. (2000). Spiritual health in residential Centers for persons with intellectual disability in Israel. A National survey. Submitted to *Journal of Intellectual Disability Research*.

Oxman, T.E., Freeman, D.H. & Manheimer, E.D. (1995). Lack of social participation or religious strength and comfort as risk factors for death after cardiac surgery in the elderly. *Psychosomatic Medicine*, 57(1), 5-15.

Porter, B. (1998). L'Arche Daybreak: An example of interfaith ministry among people with developmental disabilities. *Journal of Pastoral Care* 52(2), 157-165.

Rogers-Dulan, J. (1998). Religious connectedness among urban African American families who have a child with disabilities. *Mental Retardation*, 36(2), 91-103.

Sicher, F., Targ, E., Moore, D. & Smith, H.S. (1998). A randomized double-blind study of the effect of distant healing in a population with advanced AIDS. Report of a small scale study. *West journal of Medicine*, 169(6), 356-363.

Weisner, T.S., Beizer, L. & Stolze, L. (1991). Religion and families of children with developmental delays. *American Journal of Mental Retardation*, 95(6), 647-662.

Teaching Jewish Mentally-Retarded Youngsters Holiday Awareness Through Symbols

Varda Carmeli, MSc
Eli Carmeli, PT, PhD

SUMMARY. The purpose of the study was to test the use of various religious symbols to teach Jewish mentally-retarded youngsters enhanced familiarity with certain Jewish holidays. The participants included 8 students aged from 12-23 years old with various degrees of moderate to severe mental handicap. The study group met eight hours weekly (2 hours biweekly) for a total of 12 weeks. Four categories of questions involving nine different symbols were used. Baseline values were determined in pre- and post-testing. Results demonstrated that all students completing the study showed improvements in symbol recognition. We conclude

Varda Carmeli is Head Teacher, Neve Ram School for Children with Special Needs, Rechasim, Israel. Eli Carmeli is affiliated with the Physical Therapy Program, Sackler Faculty of Medicine, Tel Aviv University, Israel.

Address correspondence to: Dr. Eli Carmeli, Department of Physical Therapy, Sackler Faculty of Medicine, Tel Aviv University, P.O. Box 39040, Ramat Aviv 69978, Israel (E-mail: elicarmeli@hotmail.com).

The authors wish to express their deep appreciation to Ms. Fran Foreman, Central Agency for Jewish Education in Fort Lauderdale, and Dr. Harris Himot, Nova Southeastern University, Florida, for their assistance and guidance in the development and coordination of this research project.

[Haworth co-indexing entry note]: "Teaching Jewish Mentally-Retarded Youngsters Holiday Awareness Through Symbols." Carmeli, Varda, and Eli Carmeli. Co-published simultaneously in *Journal of Religion, Disability & Health* (The Haworth Pastoral Press, an imprint of The Haworth Press, Inc.) Vol. 5, No. 2/3, 2001, pp. 123-139; and: *Spirituality and Intellectual Disability: International Perspectives on the Effect of Culture and Religion on Healing Body, Mind, and Soul* (eds: William C. Gaventa, Jr. and David L. Coulter) The Haworth Pastoral Press, an imprint of The Haworth Press, Inc., 2001, pp. 123-139. Single or multiple copies of this article are available for a fee from The Haworth Document Delivery Service [1-800-342-9678, 9:00 a.m. - 5:00 p.m. (EST). E-mail address: getinfo@haworthpressinc.com].

123

that use of symbols can provide useful tools to improve communication with mentally retarded individuals. *[Article copies available for a fee from The Haworth Document Delivery Service: 1-800-342-9678. E-mail address: <getinfo@haworthpressinc.com> Website: <http://www.HaworthPress.com> © 2001 by The Haworth Press, Inc. All rights reserved.]*

KEYWORDS. Mental retardation, autistic children, teaching methods, symbols, Jewish children, religious holidays

INTRODUCTION

Several theories of early cognitive development have indicated that the use of symbols can dramatically expand intellectual horizons and facilitate communication and learning skills (Romski, Sevcik and Joyner, 1984; Uttal, Schreber and DeLoache, 1995). Children with mental retardation present a unique array of problems and display peculiar developmental patterns (Quill, 1995). Effective communication with individuals with mental retardation involves considerable effort by both the sender and the receiver of the information. A specific cognitive deficit in some children with mental retardation (Thurber and Tager-Flusberg, 1993) involves the predominance of processing abilities for visual and spatial information as compared to auditory and temporal information. Use of visual aids with individuals with mental retardation can enhance effective reception of information and responses and significantly improve interactive communication. To many of children with mental retardation, pictures and photographs have proven to be more efficient than spoken or signed forms of communication (Beadle-Brown et al., 2000). Non-verbal children with mental retardation can store the language of symbols, which can also serve as positive retrieval cues and facilitate social communication and expressive attempts (Rotholz and Berkowitz, 1989; Crossley and Gurney, 1992; Bondy and Frost, 1994; Wilkinson, Romski and Sevcik, 1994; Pierce and Schreibman, 1994).

The effects of motor and sensory stimuli on the cognitive, psychomotor and psychosocial learning skills of children with mental retardation have been reported (Abrahamsen and Mitchell, 1990; Fisher, Murray and Bundy, 1991; Gray and Garand, 1993; Newton and Hoyle, 1994). In a learning environment, sensory and motor experiences are related to several cognitive processes including attention, perception and communication.

The various Jewish holidays, representing the highlights of the Jewish year, are celebrated with specific activities and symbols, and these contribute significantly to the Jewish experience. The religious symbols serve both devotional and social functions (Gaventa, 1986) and simplify the theological and philosophical perspectives of the holiday. The symbols provide enhanced perception of specific holidays and facilitate means of expression, communication, and significance in terms of social role valorization and social inclusion. The symbols associated with the celebration of Jewish holidays include symbolic food and drinks, stories, games and various other special activities. Religious symbols are also commonly used in religion classes as teaching aids. Enhanced use of symbols should make the Jewish holidays more meaningful for children with special learning needs, however, such use of symbols to teach the Jewish life cycle to children with mental retardation has been little investigated or documented. Children with mental retardation participate in religious practices and activities, however, most public school programs for children with special needs do not emphasize religious education (but tend to maintain a neutral position). Generally, private religious schools for students with mental retardation, also do not routinely expose their students to acquisition of basic Jewish life experiences through the development of the psychomotor domain.

Students with mental retardation need to have special instruction to enable them to enjoy life more fully in their community and enable their active participation in social and religious activities. The purpose of the present study was to test the hypothesis that learning processes involving both sensory and motor integration could be improved in mentally retarded youngsters through the enhanced use of symbols. We designed a study to highlight the use of symbols as tools to improve skill acquisition in individuals with mental retardation and present some of the options that can be used by teachers and caregivers.

METHODS

The research was conducted in the framework of a special education program of the Central Agency for Jewish Education (CAJE) in South Florida. A director, with considerable expertise in special education, coordinated the class of 14 students with mental retardation, which meets regularly every Saturday and Sunday morning for Jewish religious education. Of 14 students only eight subjects were found eligible and participated in the study.

The class was taught by a team of three teachers, including an art teacher, a music teacher and a teacher of religious education. The director also trained a group of 14-20 teenagers from a local Jewish high school, who attended each class session, and provided one-on-one attention for each student with mental retardation in the program. Interaction with their teenage mentors increased the students' sense of stability and confidence. The volunteer teenagers met regularly with the assistant supervisor before each class to review methods and approaches in special education. A psychologist also volunteered her time and expertise to conduct monthly support group sessions for the parents of the students in the class and to discuss specific problems and offer possible solutions.

The student class consisted of 10 males and 4 females ($x = 15.2 \pm 3.9$ years old) with ages ranging from 12-23 years old. All students assembled in the main room where they worked individually with their own specific volunteer mentor. Six students were withdrawn from the study: two resulting from parental requests for withdrawal, two due to neurological diagnosis such as cerebral palsy, one due to scheduling for a surgical procedure, and one due to extreme retardation with strong autistic features. Hence, the total number of subjects participated in this study was eight. The study protocols received approval from the Review Committee for Studies on Human Subjects and IRB of Nova Southeastern University. Consent forms were obtained from all participant caregivers.

The study group ($n = 8$) was very heterogeneous owing to the wide variety of factors contributing to their intellectual limitation; however, all the children were diagnosed as mentally disabled with poor communication skills and limited understanding. The study group consisted of children with moderate (level II) to severe (level III) mental retardation as defined by the American Association on Mental Deficiency. These individuals have sub-average intellectual function (level II with IQ scores from 36-55 and level III with IQ scores from 20-35). Level II students are partially trainable and can learn how to communicate, although the prevalence of speech impediments is high. They usually acquire minimal academic skills, no more than those of third grade. Level III students can learn signing to supplement their limited speaking abilities, and although they can learn very basic tasks, need constant supervision in a learning environment.

A consent form with a brief introduction to the study was submitted to the parents of the students prior to a meeting where the methods and rationale of the study were explained in greater detail. The socio-economic status of the target community is considered high. Many of the parents of the students are professionals with academic degrees. The level of parental involvement in school activities and in the curriculum is very high. The parents are frequently involved in staff meetings, particularly those in which the agenda relates to the future of their child. This high degree of collaboration between parents and schoolteachers greatly improves both communication and mutual understanding.

The majority (90%) of the eight students live with their parents, whereas the rest live in group-homes as a result of their medical condition and family situation. All these students require close and constant supervision throughout the day, resulting in their almost complete dependency for life skills. In general, their expressive language skills were varied from student to student, and ranged from simple and isolated to more compound communication forms.

Additional Information About Participants

Student A was a 12-year-old girl from a single parent family following the death of her father five years previously. This girl had the lowest IQ in the study group (IQ = 36). The student constantly chewed almost every object encountered, however her oral hygiene was generally good. She cried easily without self-awareness and was mostly mute and disoriented from her surrounding. Her language skills were mainly body language, and specific gestures that she repeatedly uses.

Student B was an 18-year-old male able to speak, read, follow directions and maintain eye-contact with his teacher. The student's language skills were relatively advanced, though he tended to use a small range of topics and had some difficulty with abstract concepts.

Student C was a 24-year-old female with the highest IQ in the class (IQ = 55). This student was placed in a group home because of family problems. She was positively oriented to space, time, names and faces. Her expressive language skills through basic words were fair and comprehensible.

Student D was a 14-year-old boy with intelligence corresponding to that of an average six-year-old with short attention spans, inconsistent passiveness and lack of motivation. His communication form was mainly through language using single words or short sentences, i.e., "I want to go."

Student E was a 16-year-old boy, who usually played and worked well with toys and other objects. He was able to participate in basic conversation, with many repeated phrases.

Student F was a 12-year-old small boy, who had echolalia (repetition of words), with a reading level of third grade. He was friendly, pleasant, and fun to work with, however, he was inconsistently oriented to space, time, names, and faces,

Student G was a 16-year-old male with the second highest IQ score in the class (IQ = 52), who functioned as a third or fourth grade student. He was able to read, write and speak with others, but was restless, easily distracted and sometimes impulsive.

Student H was a 15-year-old boy (IQ = 50), who was slow, lethargic, spoke little and curtly, maintained good eye contact and responded appropriately to simple non-verbal communication.

The study took place in two buildings. One building contained three classrooms of equal dimensions providing space for classes in religion, art and music. The other building serves as a multi-purpose center used for various social and Jewish religious functions such as those of Sabbath Eve (Kabbalat Shabbat) and holidays. The interiors of the buildings were warmly decorated and clean.

A pre-test questionnaire was used to provide an initial baseline, and for later use as a source for comparison and reassessment of the participants through post-test procedures. A questionnaire with four questions was used for all eight students, for each of nine Jewish religious symbols: Rosh Hashanah (New Year) and Yom Kippur (Day of Atonement), Succot (Feast of Tabernacles), and Chanucah (Kozodoy, 1997).

The first question addressed "*What* is this?" to identify the picture, either by indicating its name, or by gesturing. The second question addressed "*When* do we use the symbol?" geared to indicate the connection between the picture and specific holidays. The third question addressed "*How* do we use the symbol?" The last question addressed "*Why* do we use the symbol?" The order of the questions followed from the simplest identification task to more integrated and analytical thinking.

A total of 12 symbols were used for this study, whereas only 9 were used in the pre- and post-tests. Twelve symbols were used during the intervening period. The three symbols used for "Rosh Hashanah" included: greeting cards, a New Year meal (including a fish head, apples and honey, pomegranate seeds) and hallah bread. The three symbols for "Yom Kippur" included: a "shofar" (curved ram's horn), prayers and the fast. The three symbols used for "Succot" included: the "succah" (tabernacle), the etrog (lemon-like citrus fruit) and "lulav" (bundle of palm branches), and the "Torah." The three symbols used for Chanucah included: a "chanukiya" (traditional candelabrum), a "dreidle" (traditional four-sided spinning-top), and potato "latkes."

The Symbols

The rationale to chose the certain symbols for this study is explained below. In the beginning of the Jewish calendar year, during the celebration of the Jewish holiday (Rosh Hashanah) they send greeting cards, and wish family and friends a happy and healthy new year. The night of the celebration consists of a Rosh Hashanah meal which incorporates special symbols, the most significant of which are eating a head of a fish, apples with honey, and the seeds of a pomegranate. The most important thing about the holiday symbols is the family gathering, to promote a message of unity and togetherness. On Rosh Hashanah it is customary to eat sweet food such as sweet hallah bread, honey cake, and fruits dipped in honey to wish that the coming year will be good and sweet. Another symbol of Rosh Hashanah and Yom Kippur is Shofar made from the curved horn of a ram. The Shofar reminds Jewish people that the Lord is present and its sounds calls upon the Lord to open the sky's gate the people prayers. Its thrilling sound is a call to action, a reminder to "pay attention" to your life. Its sounds is also an announcement that this day celebrates the creation of the world, and is a reminder of the sound at Mount Sinai before the Lord gave the Torah.

During the Jewish holiday of Sukkot, the most common symbol is the building of the Sukkah. The Torah says that after Moses led Israelis out of Egypt, they wandered for 40 years in the desert, and before they reached the Promised Land, they built huts (a Sukkah) to protect themselves from the burning sun and cold desert nights. For seven days, Jewish people bring the fruit of fine trees such as Etrog (bumpy lemon), and Lulav (bundle of palm branches) to the Sukkah. It is a reminder of the many wondrous things that grow in the earth. The Torah is the book that contains the history of the Jewish people and the Ten Commandments. Simchat Torah is the holiday when Jewish people complete the reading of the Torah and begin to read it again.

The Hanukkah menorah is a special candle holder used only during the Hunukkah holiday. In Hebrew, it is called Hanukkiah. It has holders for eight candles which according to the Jewish tradition, stands for the eight nights that the oil burned in the Temple on the first Hanukkah. The Hanukkiah has a separate holder for a ninth candle, the Shamash.

Shamash means servant or helper. The Shamash is used to light the other candles. Hannukkah is also a holiday of fun. Children play with a Dreidle. On each side of the top is a different Hebrew letter. They are the first letters of a famous Hebrew sentence, which means, "a great miracle happened there" (in Israel). On Hanukkah it is customary to eat crispy potato pancakes called Latkes. Latkes are fried in oil, to remind Jewish people of the oil that lit the holy lamp in the Temple long ago (Kozodoy, 1997).

They were several kinds of activities used in the training. Showing pictures, holding real objects, and certain activities related to the symbols: included touch, smell, taste, hear, listen, talk, sing, dance, eat, spin, etc. The intervention was carried out in different forms. Role play of the mentors, object's manipulation by students and mentors, looking, touching, holding the real objects or pictures. Hence, the sensory and motor input were integrated in the training such as lightning the chanukiya kendles, spinning the dreidle, blowing the shofar, eating latkes and so forth.

At the pre- and post-tests the students responded to the target questions through different expressive language, such as speech, manual signs and gestures. They were not trained to answer the questions in any of the interveing phases. All testers used identical pictures, short stories, and other items (e.g., greeting cards, driedle, shofar, fresh hallah bread, etrog), for the pre- and post-tests.

The grading scale and answer key was indicated on the back of each item for the tester's convenience. For the pre- and post-tests, only nine symbols were used and a maximum of 72 points was possible if the student correctly answered all 36 questions (9 symbols with 4 questions each). Points were allocated for each question as follows: two points if the answer was correct on the first try, one point if the student was cued or if the answer was partially correct, and no points for an incorrect answer. The same tester conducted both the pre-test and post-tests and recorded the data. If the student responded incorrectly to a question, the questioning was stopped (as in the pre-test).

The study lasted for 12 weeks and covered in each period questions on the first four Jewish holidays. Weekly reports were collected from the mentor of each student and data were also recorded on a narrative progress form for each participant. All data were transferred to spreadsheets, which allowed their users to re-code the data to a progress form. Three categories of answers were recorded (correct, partially correct, and incorrect). The analysis program included instructions to code the categories for symbols 1 through 9 (2 points for correct answers, 1 point for partially correct answers, and 0 points for incorrect answers or failure to respond). During the recording process, a preliminary analysis of data for all questions was undertaken to determine specific features, such as frequency and percentages for each category. A post-test with a similar format was conducted during week 12.

The Intervening Period

The links between sensory input and motor output for basic skill acquisition have been previously reported (Higgins, 1991; Schmidt, 1991). Training and learning processes are facilitated by an integrated sensory and motor approach. The students met for twelve consecutive Saturdays and Sundays, for a total of eight hours a week. Only those symbols relevant to the actual holiday were practiced. In between the pre- and post-tests, each student was exposed to the selected symbols, progressively one at the time, for a total of 12 symbols, coinciding with the Jewish holidays occurring between September and the end of December. Each session lasted four hours. Each symbol has its own distinctive features. The symbols differ from each other according to their specific shape, color, sound, weight, smell, etc. Sensory input for each symbol involved the use of a wide range of senses (touch, vision, smell, hearing, and taste). In addition, the teacher related short stories, with special emphasis on the symbols and their special features (e.g., why and how the "dreidle" spins; the sounds of the "shofar"; the smell of the "latkes").

Statistical Analysis

All data were analyzed with SPSS 7.2 for Windows 97. Paired or correlated *t* tests were used to compare the differences between baseline values of pre- and post-tests. One-group pre- and post-test design is a quasi-experimental design commonly used in clinical research. The critical values for statistical significance were assumed at an alpha level < 0.05.

Selection, Training and Reliability of Testers

Two teachers were selected to administer the questionnaire in addition to the researcher, who served as an independent observer during the pre- and post-tests. The researcher explained the study to the teachers, and trained them in administration of the questions, data collection and use of the spreadsheet form. The reliability and validity of the symbolic questions was then tested in a group of 23 regular schoolchildren without mental handicaps (mean age 13.4 ± 3.6) and was shown to be very high (K = 0.98; p < 0.05). Inter-rater reliability was addressed with each tester in a different room randomly testing two students in a 1:1 session. Each tester used the same data-collection system (i.e., the questionnaire including the four questions for nine symbols). The level of agreement between the tester was calculated by dividing the number of agreements on the marked and completed questionnaire by the total number of agreements plus disagreements and multiplying by 100, resulting in a reliability ranging from 96% to 98%. Inter-tester reliability (Kappa statistics) was found to be high (K = 0.94; p < 0.05). We are aware that testing validity and reliability in another group than the target group does not automatically mean that the instrument is working the same when we used it in the study. This is particularly true when few of the students with mental retardation were not able to respond with intelligible spoken language as the other group. Yet, we believe that validity and reliability method we used and the high score we got, allowed us to predict a true positive of the outcomes. In the intervening period, the teachers and volunteers implemented specific procedures in order to expose all the students to standard treatment protocols.

RESULTS

All of the students worked well with the four categories of the nine symbols, though some difficulties were noted in particular with the fourth "*why?*" question. The pre-and post-tests consisted of four identical questions and nine identical symbols. In both tests, the questioning stopped once the student had made two consecutive error responses or if the student totally neglected the question or ignored the tester.

Tables 1 and 2 display the pre-and post-test responses (values in points) whereas Table 3 displays the percentage differences between the two tests involving nine symbols. The results indicated that all students (but student C and H) showed some improvement when they answered the first symbol question, ("*What?*"). Six students recognized all nine symbols.

Student A was only able to recognize two of the nine symbols (the dreidel and the Torah). During the post-test the student was able to match picture to picture when the tester directly asked her, which is a non-significant improvement of 5.5%. The student received four points out of 18 possible points in the post-test questions. Student D improved significantly by 22.2% and recognized eight of the nine symbols (except the "lulav"). In the post-test he received 16 out of 18 points. Students B, E, and G showed significant improvements, 16.7%, 39% and 11% respectively on the *"What?"* question. Student B for the second *"When?"* question answered four more questions correctly and improved significantly by 39%. Student C answered one more question with non-significant improvement. Students E, F, and H significantly improved and were able to answer six, four, and six more of the "When?" questions, respectively. Student G only slightly improved by 5.6% and was able to answer all nine "When?" questions. The results of the "When?" questions indicated that the most significant improvement occurred among those students who did relatively poorly on the pre-test. The results of the third and the fourth questions, "How?" and "Why" the symbol was used are demonstrated in Tables 1, 2, and 3. The poorest improvement was associated with the fourth question.

DISCUSSION

The aim of the study was to enhance familiarity with religious symbols. This purpose was relatively accomplished, and most students were able to identify the symbols and answer the questions about them. Students having communication deficiencies make learning processes extremely difficult (Schaeffer, 1980; Lloyd and Karlan, 1984) and in order to have a learning process in class, special teaching methods need to be adopted by teachers and volunteers (Bonvillian and Miller, 1995). This may involve special organization of the teaching environment, and enhanced use of sensory and motor stimulation in order to improve attention levels and increase learning motivation (Tennyson and Cocchiarella, 1986). The teaching methods need to be adjusted to student's cognition and intelligence levels. Enhanced use of symbols can be used as communication tools with children with mental retardation, especially those symbols involving the senses of touch, taste, smell, vision and hearing (Adams, 1987), and perhaps facilitate prolonged retention. The spiritual needs of the students to practice Judaism through religious symbols is important. By recognizing and understanding the symbol's significance, in terms of the child's experience (i.e., good time, exciting, unusual food) he or she practices a spiritual experience.

Students with mental retardation need the opportunity to enjoy religious activities and holidays. This would set their scene for including

TABLE 1. Pre-test baseline responses of participants (n = 8) to nine symbols. Values are points

Student Symbol	Question	A	B	C	D	E	F	G	H
1. Dreidel	What?	0	2	2	2	2	2	2	2
	When?	0	2	2	0	2	2	2	2
	How?	0	1	2	0	2	1	2	2
	Why?	0	0	1	0	1	0	2	1
2. New Year Card	What?	0	1	2	2	0	1	2	2
	When?	0	0	2	0	0	1	2	2
	How?	0	1	2	0	0	1	2	2
	Why?	0	0	2	0	0	0	0	0
3. Torah	What?	0	2	2	0	1	2	2	2
	When?	0	2	1	0	1	2	2	0
	How?	0	2	2	0	0	0	2	1
	Why?	0	0	0	0	0	0	0	0
4. Chanukia	What?	0	2	2	0	1	2	2	2
	When?	0	0	2	0	2	0	2	1
	How?	0	0	2	0	1	0	2	1
	Why?	0	0	2	0	0	0	0	0
5. Shofar	What?	0	1	2	0	2	2	2	2
	When?	0	2	2	0	0	2	2	1
	How?	0	2	2	0	1	1	2	1
	Why?	0	0	1	0	0	0	1	0
6. Succah	What?	0	1	2	0	2	2	2	2
	When?	0	1	2	0	0	1	2	2
	How?	0	0	2	0	0	0	2	0
	Why?	0	0	0	0	0	0	0	0
7. Latkes	What?	0	2	2	0	1	2	1	2
	When?	0	0	2	0	2	0	2	1
	How?	0	2	2	0	2	0	2	1
	Why?	0	0	2	0	0	0	0	0
8. Apple and Honey	What?	0	2	2	0	2	2	2	2
	When?	0	2	2	0	0	2	2	1
	How?	0	2	2	0	2	0	2	1
	Why?	0	0	2	0	0	0	1	0
9. Lulav	What?	0	2	2	0	0	2	2	2
	When?	0	2	2	0	0	2	1	1
	How?	0	0	2	0	0	0	2	2
	Why?	0	0	0	0	0	0	0	0
Total		0	36	63	4	27	33	55	41

TABLE 2. Post-test baseline responses of participants (n = 8) to nine symbols. Values are points

Student Symbol	Question	A	B	C	D	E	F	G	H
1. Dreidel	What?	2	2	2	2	2	2	2	2
	When?	0	2	2	2	2	2	2	2
	How?	0	2	2	2	2	2	2	2
	Why?	0	2	2	0	1	1	2	2
2. New Year Card	What?	0	2	2	2	2	2	2	2
	When?	0	2	2	2	2	2	2	2
	How?	0	2	2	0	2	2	2	2
	Why?	0	1	2	0	0	1	2	2
3. Torah	What?	2	2	2	2	2	2	2	2
	When?	0	2	2	0	2	2	2	2
	How?	0	2	2	0	0	2	2	2
	Why?	0	0	1	0	0	0	0	0
4. Chanukia	What?	0	2	2	2	2	2	2	2
	When?	0	2	2	0	2	2	2	2
	How?	0	2	2	0	2	2	2	2
	Why?	0	0	2	0	0	0	0	0
5. Shofar	What?	0	2	2	2	2	2	2	2
	When?	0	2	2	0	2	2	2	2
	How?	0	2	2	0	2	2	2	2
	Why?	0	0	1	0	0	0	2	0
6. Succah	What?	0	2	2	2	2	2	2	2
	When?	0	2	2	0	2	2	2	2
	How?	0	2	2	0	1	1	2	2
	Why?	0	0	1	0	0	0	2	0
7. Latkes	What?	0	2	2	2	2	2	2	2
	When?	0	2	2	0	2	2	2	2
	How?	0	2	2	0	2	2	2	2
	Why?	0	0	2	0	0	0	2	0
8. Apple and Honey	What?	0	2	2	2	2	2	2	2
	When?	0	2	2	2	2	2	2	2
	How?	0	2	2	0	2	2	2	2
	Why?	0	2	2	0	0	0	2	2
9. Lulav	What?	0	2	2	0	2	2	2	2
	When?	0	2	2	0	2	2	2	2
	How?	0	2	2	0	0	2	2	2
	Why?	0	0	1	0	0	0	0	0
Total		4	59	68	20	50	55	66	60

TABLE 3. Percentage (%) of participants' responses to four categories of questions (n = 8).

Question Category	What?		When?		How?		Why?		Total		t test
Student	Pre	Post	Pre	Post	Pre	Post	Pre	Post	Pre	Post	p value
A	0	- 22.2	0	- 0	0	- 0	0	- 0	0	- 5.5	N.S.
B	83.3 -	100	61.1 -	100	55.5 -	100	0	- 27	50	- 82.0	p < 0.05
C	100 -	100	94.4 -	100	100	- 100	55.5 -	77.7	87.5 -	94.4	p < 0.05
D	22.2 -	88.8	0	- 11.1	0	- 11.1	0	- 0	5.5	- 27.7	p < 0.001
E	61.1 -	100	38.8 -	100	44.4 -	61.1	5.5	- 16.6	37.5 -	69.4	p < 0.001
F	100 -	100	66.6 -	100	16.6 -	94.4	0	- 11.1	48.8 -	76.3	p < 0.05
G	88.8 -	100	94.4 -	100	100	- 100	22.2 -	66.6	76.3 -	91.6	p < 0.02
H	100 -	100	61.1 -	100	61.1 -	100	5.5	- 33.3	56.9 -	83.3	p < 0.02

Values are %; differences between pre-test and post-test were assessed using correlated t test, with critical value assumed p < 0.05. N.S. = non-significant

intellectually impaired individuals as part of the wider Jewish community and enhancing their opportunities for involvement. Improving Jewish education in students with mental retardation presents a major challenge. Understanding the holiday's symbols can lead to increased awareness and participation of the students in the celebrations. The familiarity with the symbols does not necessarily mean that the students with mental retardation know anything about the meaning of the symbols in the real setting (i.e., in a ceremony at the holiday) and how functional their learned skills are. Students who are mentally handicapped have problems with generalizing learned skills to a functional use. Indeed, the ultimate goal of a new skill acquisition is to implement and to reflect it in a meaningful manner. Higgins 1991 says that the ability to do it is a slow, progressively modified process that should be suited and adapted by each child. Moreover, integration and generalization of new knowledge may not be straight-forward, or immediately applicated, yet it provides an opportunity for this process and potential for important new growth.

Using the same questions for each symbol in the study helped evaluate the level of knowledge and awareness of each individual, and identify their specific learning needs. The four questions were not oriented toward specific disabilities but rather toward specific situations, which can be used for future implementation and follow-up assessment.

We considered two possible explanations regarding the data relating to the student's ease in symbol recognition (the questions "What?", "When?", and "How?"), and their difficulties in analyzing the use of the symbols (the "Why?" question). The first explanation is that the ease of recognition resulted from the weekly repetition of the symbols. The role of repetition in acquisition and retention of knowledge has not been investigated extensively. Sensory and motor integration, accompanied by cognitive processes, is a major factor affecting retention and learning of symbols. Every time a specific symbol is presented it makes the student draw upon previous experience and enhances memory retention. A further possible explanation is that although the students were capable of recognizing and answering the first three questions concerning each symbol, the majority of them could not answer the more demanding "Why?" question due to limited mental competence and lack of overall cognitive integration. The effects of past experience appear to be very important elements influencing cognitive integration for retention and future recall. Whereas each religious symbol is based on traditions amassed over generations, such a collection of religious knowledge and experience is lacking in individuals with mental retardation. The results clearly show, nonetheless, that considerable learning can occur even in the absence of complete cognitive integration. Collectively, the methods and the conditions under which the study was conducted could affect these two explanations. Individuals with mental retardation are mainly visual thinkers and hands-on learners, and best learn when visual and sensorimotor methods are involved. Effective learning requires more than just repetition. Although repetition may benefit immediate performance, there may be poor retention. Consequently, long-term retention in such cases requires modifying the teaching techniques (Parson, Reid and Green, 1996).

A future study for teaching the religious symbols should extend the scope of this research in order to compare other behavioral approaches, such as discrete trial-and-error and incidental teaching. The pre- and post-tests were done without withdrawal periods. Such a period can show long term retention. A future study could teach children with mental retardation and autistic students the specific religious items (e.g., the chanukiya), and use picture symbols for each of the items for communication purposes, and then use them functionally in a daily schedule (e.g., lighting the chanukiya during Chanukah).

In conclusion, our study has shown that the use of religious symbols can increase cognition and perception in young Jewish students with mental disabilities and lead to their enhanced appreciation of the Jewish holidays and increased participation in these special occasions. We have highlighted various options for teachers and caregivers in the potential benefits of using symbols in teaching individuals with mental retardation, leading to improved skill acquisition and learning.

REFERENCES

Abrahamsen, E. P., & Mitchell, J. R. (1990). Communication and sensorimotor functioning in children with autism. *J Autism Devel Disord* 20: 75-85.

Adams, J. A. (1987). Historical review and appraisal of research on the learning, retention, and transfer of human motor skills. *Psychol Bull* 101: 41-74.

Beadle-Brwon, J., Murphy, G., Wing, L., Gould, J., Shah, A., & Holmes, N. (2000). Changes in skills for people with intellectual disability. *Journal of Intellectual Disability Research*. 44: 12-24.

Bondy, A, & Frost, L. (1994). The picture exchange communication system. *Focus on Autism Behavior* 9: 1-19.

Bonvillian, R. D., & Miller, A. J. (1995). Everything old is new again: Observation from nineteenth century about sign communication training with mentally retarded children. *Sign Communication Training* 88: 245-253.

Crossley, R., & Gurney, J. R. (1992). Getting the words out: Facilitated communication training. *Topics in Language Dis* 12: 29-45.

Fisher, A. G., Murray, E. A., & Bundy, A. C. (1991). Combining sensory integration with behavioral theory for child with mental retardation. In: Sensory Integration: Theory and Practice, pp 375-378. Philadelphia, F. A. Davis.

Gaventa, W. C. (1986). Religious ministries and services with adults with developmental disabilities. In: J. A. Summers (Ed), The Right to Grow Up., pp 191-226. Baltimore. P. H. Brokkes.

Gray, C. A., & Garand, J. D. (1993). Social stories: Improving responses of students with autism with accurate social information. *Focus on Autistic Behavior* 8: 1-10.

Higgins, S. (1991). Motor skill acquisition. *Physical Therapy* 71: 123-139.

Kozodoy, R.L. (1997). The book of Jewish holidays. West Orange, NJ, Behrman House.

Lloyd, L. L., & Karlan, G. R. (1984). Non-speech communication symbols and systems: Where have we been and where are we going. *J Mental Defic Res* 28: 3-20.

Newton, S., & Hoyle, E. (1994). Culture and survival: The role of symbols in improving the quality of a comprehensive school. *School Organization* 14: 309-319.

Parson, M. B., Reid, D. H., & Green, C. W. (1996). Training basic teaching skills to community children: A case study. *Language, Speech and Hearing Services in Schools* 19: 128-143.

Pierce, K., Schreibman, L. (1994). Teaching daily living skills to children with autism in unsupervised settings through pictorial self-management. *J Appl Behavior Analysis* 27: 471-481.

Quill, K. A. (1995). Visually cues instruction for children with autism and pervasive developmental disorders. *Focus on Autistic Behavior* 10: 10-20.

Romski, M. A., Sevcik, R. A., & Joyner, S. E. (1984). Non-speech communication systems: Implications for language intervention with mentally retarded children. *Topics in Language Disorders* 3: 66-81.

Rotholz, D. A., & Berkowitz, S. F. (1989). Functionality of two modes of communication in the community by students with developmental disabilities: A comparison of signing and communication books. *J Assoc for Persons with Severe Handicaps* 14: 227-233.

Schaeffer, B. (1980). Teaching signed speech to non-verbal children. *Sign Language Studies* 26: 29-63.

Schmidt, R. A (1991). Motor learning principles. In: Contemporary Management of Motor Control Problems. Foundation APTA (ed.), Chapter 7 pp. 49-63, Virginia, USA.

Tennyson, R. D., & Cocchiarella, M. J. (1986). An empirically based instructional design theory of teaching concept. *Rev Edu Res* 56: 40-71.

Thurber, C., & Tager-Flusberg, H. (1993). Pauses in the narratives produced by autistic, mentally retarded, and normal children as an index of cognitive demand. *J Autism Develop Disord* 23: 309-322.

Uttal, D., Schreiber, J. C., & DeLoache, J. S. (1995). Waiting to use a symbol: The effects of delay on children's use of models. *Child Develop* 66: 1875-1889.

Wilkinson, K. M., Romski, M. A., & Sevcik, R. A. (1994). Emergence of visual graphic symbol combinations by youth with moderate or severe mental retardation. *J Speech Hearing Res* 37: 883-895.

IV. FROM THEORY AND THEOLOGY TO PRACTICE: CREATIVE WAYS OF FACILITATING SPIRITUAL HEALTH

Liturgical Celebration with People with a Severe Mental Disability: Giving the Gospel Hands and Feet

Anja Vogelzang, Drs

SUMMARY. Anja Vogelzang, a Chaplain at De Hartenberg, a residential facility in the Netherlands, describes the rationale and process for a worship service conducted with people with severe mental disabilities and multiple disabilities. She focuses on ways to build celebration and community. *[Article copies available for a fee from The Haworth Document Delivery Service: 1-800-342-9678. E-mail address: <getinfo@haworthpressinc.com> Website: <http://www.HaworthPress.com> © 2001 by The Haworth Press, Inc. All rights reserved.]*

Anja Vogelzang is Chaplain at De Hartenberg in the Netherlands.
Address correspondence to: Anja Vogelzang, Alascholversingel 3, 6883 BA, VELP, Netherlands (E-mail: anja.vogelzang@hotmail.com).

[Haworth co-indexing entry note]: "Liturgical Celebration with People with a Severe Mental Disability: Giving the Gospel Hands and Feet." Vogelzang, Anja. Co-published simultaneously in *Journal of Religion, Disability & Health* (The Haworth Pastoral Press, an imprint of The Haworth Press, Inc.) Vol. 5, No. 2/3, 2001, pp. 141-146; and: *Spirituality and Intellectual Disability: International Perspectives on the Effect of Culture and Religion on Healing Body, Mind, and Soul* (eds: William C. Gaventa, Jr. and David L. Coulter) The Haworth Pastoral Press, an imprint of The Haworth Press, Inc., 2001, pp. 141-146. Single or multiple copies of this article are available for a fee from The Haworth Document Delivery Service [1-800-342-9678, 9:00 a.m. - 5:00 p.m. (EST). E-mail address: getinfo@haworthpressinc.com].

141

KEYWORDS. Worship, severe mental disability, celebration, community, gospel, music

Create here a new force of imagination
Give language and music to our dreams
Give voice to what remained obscure
Let here Your Kingdom come

In dealing with pastoral care for people with a severe mental disability, we often discover the fundamental problem is that the normal ways of working with people in catechises and other forms of pastoral teaching are not possible.

The communication of the Gospel is normally done in ways strongly characterised by using words. We often tell a (Bible) story, sing together and pray together. But this is meaningful to human beings that understand language and are themselves capable of using verbal ways of communication. They can 'live through' a story and thus experience God in their lives and share it with others. However, human beings with nearly no understanding or without any understanding of words are not properly taken into account.

Together with care-assistants of people with a severe mental disability, we have searched for pastoral ways and means of relating to them. And we are confident we have found a good method in the form of a special way of liturgical celebration.

In these celebrations, language in the form of the 'spoken word' is less important. We celebrate our being together and, also, that everyone is a meaningful part of our community and that our presence on earth is a good thing. We celebrate our being created by God as human beings, created in His image. Conceptions such as love, sharing and caring are important. If we want people with a severe mental disability to experience these biblical conceptions, we have to create conditions in which the Gospel has been given 'hands' and 'feet.'

So how does it work, such a celebration?

THE PREPARATIONS

Before we start with the celebration, we prepare a small liturgical room. The curtains and sun-blinds are closed to darken the room a little. Low lighting and special effect lighting is used. If necessary, a smaller room is created with the help of screens. The chairs and cushions are arranged so as to leave enough space for the wheelchairs. Some sheepskin-mats are put in a circle on the floor. The big Easter-candle is put on the liturgical table. Next to it, some little candles are placed, together with the heather, the display for the etheric oil, the songbooks, and some images and objects to stimulate the senses. Seasonal flowers decorate the liturgical table.

In the kitchen-corner, coffee, tea and yoghurt-drinks are prepared. Hot water bottles are filled with hot water and put on the central heating, to keep warm and distributed to those participants who like them. If there is no live music, a selection of recorded music can be used while participants are arriving and during the celebration. It is important for the conductor to take enough time for these preparations, because one of the mean features of those liturgical celebrations is its relaxed atmosphere. If you are still arranging or preparing things during the celebration, this can disturb the participants unnecessarily. At the arranged time the participants, people with a severe disability and their assistants, gather together to the liturgical room. The group usually contains 8-12 people.

An important feature is the intense participation of all individuals. We emphasize the importance of a sufficient number of assistants in order to provide personal attention to everybody. This is an essential element, for by being there, by reaching out to someone else, through human warmth, attention and intimacy, we experience God's love and care in our midst. Once everybody has been seated in the circle, the liturgical celebration can start.

THE CELEBRATION

At the beginning of the celebration the conductor goes to every participant with a triangle while singing some lines. The high, thin sound of the instrument and the singing voice often arouse a reaction in the participants. Everybody is called by his name and told that the celebration is beginning.

With the assistants, we sing the traditional songs of the beginning: "We welcome you all" and "Come yea in the circle." Sometimes a short, simple prayer is said. Now the Easter candle is lit and we pronounce the name of Jesus, who is risen and is the Light of the world for us. Then we sing the song of the Light. Thereupon, little candles for everyone present are lit from the Easter candle. With these burning candles the conductor visits every participant and sings a song of welcome: "hello, . . . , hello . . . , we're glad that you are with us!" The assistants also are welcomed with the lighting of a candle. When everybody has a candle and these are put near the Easter candle, we sing a song about small candles near the great Light.

Subsequently we sing some well-known songs. Most participants cannot sing or are only partly capable of singing these songs. Nevertheless, our experience has shown that it is good that songs are sung: people recognize a song they like, enjoy the combination of music and human voices and/or enjoy the personal attention that is given during the singing. The singing together contributes to a special atmosphere. After the singing the lights are put out. Now only the Easter candle, the small candles and the black-light are shining. The projector illumines liquid, throwing soft flowing colours on the wall.

We listen to music, if possible live, e.g., piano, harp or guitar. Especially stringed instruments can create an intimate atmosphere, but flute music is also very suitable. When we use recorded music, a choir or peaceful instrumental (religious) music is chosen. In the meantime, we aim our attention to the participants. By using the human voice, mime or physical touch, we try to relate to people that want to relate. Sometimes people spontaneously come and sit on our laps or lean on us. We use objects like soft cloths, feather boas, cuddly toys, toys for touching and musical instruments to help contact.

So, too, by way of personal contact, we try to share warmth and intimacy. And we hope and believe that by doing this, for a brief moment God becomes tangible.

This part is the core of the celebration and lasts about 10 or 15 minutes. Much depends on the needs of a certain group and on the atmosphere that exists on the spot. Then this part of the celebration is stopped. Slowly the volume of the music is turned down, more light is put on and the 'liquid-projector' is turned off.

We sing some songs. Sometimes a blessing is pronounced or sung. Thereupon, the candles are blown out and, again, we relate to every participant. In closing, we eat or drink a little together. An atmosphere of peace, coziness and relaxation is created. We talk together quietly and assist the participants that want to communicate. After about 45 minutes, the celebration is over. The Easter candle is blown out. Everybody—if necessary—is assisted in putting on his coat or getting back into the wheelchair. In two weeks time, this group may return for another celebration.

WHAT MAKES THESE LITURGICAL CELEBRATIONS DIFFERENT?

Often, we are asked the question about the difference in this liturgical celebration, wherein we stimulate the senses, and other sensorial meetings performed by those occupied in organising day activities for people with severe mental disabilities. One of the differences is in our 'objects,' our symbols. First, there is the important role of the Easter candle and the little lights around it. And, furthermore, the choice of our music is different. There is also the circle, wherein we sit and perform the activities, which emphasizes the joint relation as a group.

The most important difference, however, is in the intention, the reason why we celebrate. In liturgical celebration everything we do and all things we use are directed to one objective: to give people the possibility to be together, to experience God's love and our being cared for by His love in their own way. Liturgical celebration is an action of faith. And this leads us to the core of the matter: faith in the love of God is all about community and doing things together.

TO GIVE 'HANDS' AND 'FEET' TO THE GOSPEL

By celebrating together, we are put into action and discover our participation in the great secret of light and life. The story of our life and the life of people around us can be characterized by pain, sorrow and imperfection. By sharing the secret of the Light, which shines into, our often senseless, lives, we partake in God's history with men and, through this, our lives can find new meaning.

We celebrate that we are not alone. We celebrate the promise contained in the name of God: "I will be!" We are protected in this Name. And as children of God, we carry the image of His Name; we are created in His Image, as the Scripture tells us.

This gives us meaning and in it we are all the same. In God's Name we are called to be common partners, because only in community will we be wholly human. In as much as God is a God that relates, we too can only fully develop as human beings when we relate to others. Self-identity is only acquired through other people. Self-identity is only fostered through the way we relate to others as unique persons.

Attributes such as knowledge and skill are no longer important. Meaning something to somebody has to do with love; the other person—in seeing him or her—and it will awaken love in you!

The meaning of celebration therefore becomes meeting someone else in his own capacity. And this capacity in the end becomes communal. And so we share in God's love, an experience we often cannot describe in words. The circle we create during the celebration is a symbol of community.

Where somebody is left outside, community no longer exists. The ambiguity of our existence is featured by the constant disruptions in community. We, ourselves, are outside community or we shut off others from it. We live in an imperfect world; our existence is 'not-yet' perfect. To celebrate is to live in the expectation of the true community, which is promised to us by Scripture. By celebrating we anticipate the fulfillment of this promise in faith, hope and love. Our imagination is nurtured and carries us into the Great Story of God and men. We do as Jesus did; give hands and feet to the secret of the Word, putting our trust on the Light that is, was and will be.

The Benefits of Jewish Mourning Rituals for the Grieving Individual with Intellectual Disabilities

Shlomo Kessel, MA
Joav Merrick, MD, DMSc

SUMMARY. Death in any family is a traumatic event that disturbs the regular course of life. The present population of persons with intellectual disability is most probably the first generation of aging people with intellectual disabilities ever living. The increase in their life expectancy makes the possibility of experiences with separation, death and mourning a new reality for this population. Parents or siblings are passing away and the person with intellectual disability continues to live. This presentation is a review of the literature of mourning with special focus on Jewish mourning rituals related to persons with intellectual disability drawn from our experiences with this population in residential care in Israel. *[Article copies available for a fee from The Haworth Document Delivery Service: 1-800-342-9678. E-mail address: <getinfo@haworthpressinc.com> Website: <http://www.HaworthPress.com> © 2001 by The Haworth Press, Inc. All rights reserved.]*

Shlomo Kessel is Director of Neve Natoa Residential Center, Box 93, IL-38110 Hadera, Israel (E-mail: skessel@internet-zahav.net). Joav Merrick is Medical Director of the Division for Mental Retardation, Ministry of Labour and Social Affairs, P.O. Box 1260, IL-91012 Jerusalem, Israel (E-mail: jmerrick@ aquanet.co.il).

[Haworth co-indexing entry note]: "The Benefits of Jewish Mourning Rituals for the Grieving Individual with Intellectual Disabilities." Kessel, Shlomo and Joav Merrick. Co-published simultaneously in *Journal of Religion, Disability & Health* (The Haworth Pastoral Press, an imprint of The Haworth Press, Inc.) Vol. 5, No. 2/3, 2001, pp. 147-156; and: *Spirituality and Intellectual Disability: International Perspectives on the Effect of Culture and Religion on Healing Body, Mind, and Soul* (eds: William C. Gaventa, Jr. and David L. Coulter) The Haworth Pastoral Press, an imprint of The Haworth Press, Inc., 2001, pp. 147-156. Single or multiple copies of this article are available for a fee from The Haworth Document Delivery Service [1-800-342-9678, 9:00 a.m. - 5:00 p.m. (EST). E-mail address: getinfo@haworthpressinc.com].

147

KEYWORDS. Grief, bereavement, mourning, death, Jewish mourning rituals, intellectual disability, Israel

The encounter and the need to deal with life transitions and their accompanying losses and grief, are common phenomena in the lives of aging people (Kloeppel & Hollins, 1989). As life expectancy in the western world rapidly increases, individuals are undergoing more experiences that include bereavement.

Death in the family is a traumatic event that disturbs the regular course of life. Aging should therefore be seen as an internal developmental process that sets demands on the person to cope with distress caused by the loss of significant others. Bereavement includes the process of coping and the various reactions experienced by the individual who has lost a loved one. We refer to behavioral, cognitive and emotional changes. Often the bereavement is expressed in the form of behaviors that demonstrate the person's grief as the result of his having been separated from a loved one, a treasured possession or his familiar environment (Harper & Wadsworth, 1993).

Older individuals experience bereavement from various sources. The death of parents, family members and other loved ones, while being the best recognized source, is only one of the reasons. The aging person may feel grief and sorrow as the result of a gradual decline of his or her physical or cognitive abilities. Functional decline is a well-known and normative phenomenon of the aging process, however it is still difficult for the individual to accept the loss of his abilities (Ludlow, 1999).

AGING ADULTS WITH INTELLECTUAL DISABILITIES– AN EMERGING POPULATION

One of the important consequences of the progress of medical technology and improved social awareness in the twentieth century, is the increasing life span of people with intellectual and other developmental disabilities (Hollins & Esterhuyzen, 1997). In the past the majority of individuals with intellectual disability died at a young age and, therefore, never underwent the aging process. When compared to people without disabilities, the aging process creates many unique and complex tensions for aging individuals with mental retardation, mainly as a result of their often being dependent on others for daily support. In addition, they may demonstrate cognitive difficulties and deficient communicative skills. The situation may be worsened as the result of discriminatory social attitudes that impede and limit the access of aging individuals with intellectual disabilities to information and support (Ludlow, 1999).

The increase in the life expectancy of people with intellectual disabilities is a "two edged sword." These individuals enjoy the blessing of a long and healthy life. However, they also experience the pain and sorrow that often, accompanies the aging process. More people now have contact with separation, death and mourning. Today, we witness an emerging phenomenon where traditional care providers, such as parents or siblings, are passing away, while their aging relatives with intellectual disabilities whom they supported, are still living—sometimes with nobody left to care for them.

The issues of loss and bereavement are familiar issues to those who are involved with adults who have developmental disabilities. Unfortunately, there is little recognition of the impact of loss on this population.

THE POPULATION OF PERSONS WITH INTELLECTUAL DISABILITY IN RESIDENTIAL CARE IN ISRAEL

From the establishment of the modern State of Israel in 1948 until 1962, the Ministry of Welfare was responsible for the care of persons with mental retardation, developmental disability or intellectual disability (in this article the term intellectual disability will be used). In 1962, the Division for the Mentally Retarded (DMR) was established under the Ministry of Labour and Social Affairs with the responsibility for the assessment, treatment and rehabilitation of persons with an intellectual disability (ID).

Today in Israel there is a total population of 6,037,000 persons. The DMR is in contact with close to 20,000 persons (all ages). Residential care is provided to about 6,000 persons in 53 residential centers all over the country. Another 1,700 persons are provided residential care in hostels or group homes in the community in about another 50 places. The other 12,300 persons are served with day-care kindergarten, day-treatment centers, sheltered workshops or integrated care in the community.

The age distribution of 6,022 persons with ID in residential centers from 1998 is presented in Table 1 and the level of mental retardation presented in Table 2. There were nine government, 32 private and 12 public centers with a mean of 113.62 persons in each institution (range 22-398). It is worth noting that the total expenditure is provided by the

TABLE 1. The population of persons with intellectual disability in institutions in Israel 1998.

Age in Years	Males	Females	Total	Percent
0-10	125	118	243	4.05
11-18	414	316	730	12.12
19-45	2,099	1,533	3,632	60.31
46-60	600	624	1,224	20.32
> 61	100	93	193	3.20
Total	3,338	2,684	6,022	100.00

TABLE 2. The level of mental retardation (MR) the population of persons with intellectual disability in institutions in Israel 1998. Mild MR: IQ 55-70, moderate: IQ 35-54, severe: IQ 20-34 and profound: IQ < 20. Other are three persons, who historically were placed in institutions for other reasons and prefered to stay on, because they regarded the institution as their home.

Age in Years	Mild	Moderate	Severe	Profound	Other	Total	Percent
0-10	2	25	44	172	0	243	4.05
11-18	25	194	284	226	1	730	12.12
19-45	308	1,481	1,133	709	1	3,632	60.31
46-60	142	660	237	184	1	1,224	20.32
> 61	15	122	47	9	0	193	3.20
Total	492	2,482	1,745	1,300	3	6,022	100.00

government, which also runs the government residential centers; whereas the private and public centers are with their own administration, but provided for in the budget, the clients, and supervised by the government.

The Natoa Residential Center is one of the private residential centers affiliated with the Ministry of Labour and Social Affairs. It has a population of 166 persons (109 males and 57 females), 84 in the ages of 19-45 years, 78 aged 46-60 years, and four over the age of 61 years. This residential center provided the study population for this presentation.

BEREAVEMENT AND PERSONS
WITH INTELLECTUAL DISABILITIES

Usually within this group, the definition of loss tends to be a traditional one (i.e., death) rather than inclusive of the whole range of losses that an individual with developmental disabilities may experience. Individuals with intellectual and other developmental disabilities experience losses stemming from different sources. In addition to the "traditional" parting from a loved one who has passed on, they experience loss resulting from the replacement of a principal caregiver, from being arbitrarily transferred from one service or residential program to another and, similar to all aging individuals, from the loss of physical and cognitive functioning (Stoddart & McDonnell, 1999).

Even when there is recognition of the impact of losses on the individual, people who make up the person's support system may be unsure of how to address losses. The loss of a significant relationship has an overpowering and often devastating effect on the lives of the individuals with intellectual disabilities, their families and the services supporting them (Stoddart & McDonnell, 1999).

In many cases, when the passing of a close relative of an individual with intellectual disabilities occurs, he is prevented from participating in the funeral. Often, the individual with disabilities is not told of the death for weeks or months after it has happened, or even not told at all. Thus, the basic rights of these individuals are seriously violated and, as professionals, we should be profoundly disturbed by this phenomenon and search for appropriate solutions.

Harper and Wadworth (1993) stress the tendency to see both mental retardation (intellectual disabilities) and death as taboo subjects in western society. For many, death is seen as "distant and unexplored territory." For most of our lives we live under the illusion that life is endless and that death is something that happens to others (Moise, 1978). For this reason, many families and professionals are unprepared to handle death and feel unqualified to deal with the task of breaking the tragic news to the person with intellectual disabilities. They may mistakenly believe that these individuals do not possess the capacity to understand the implications of death (e.g., that it is final, that it is not their fault), that they are unable to form or experience significant relationships, or that they are unable to feel sorrow or grief for the loved person who has died (Stoddart & McDonnell, 1999). Moreover, there are those who believe that it is better to divert the person's attention from the memory of the person who has passed away and, thus, help him to forget. Many erroneously feel that the person with intellectual disabilities has had a difficult and distressful life and should be protected from further pain and sorrow.

While the intentions of the family members and others may be noble, it is our opinion that this form of over-protectiveness is misplaced and, indeed, violates the basic human rights of the person involved. Many professionals claim that excluding the person with intellectual disabilities from the bereavement process, is the cause of irreparable psychological harm and injury to his spiritual well-being (Deutsch, 1985; Seltzer, 1985). The lack of an appropriate opportunity to express his previous losses, may trigger a delayed and exaggerated grief response in the person with intellectual disabilities who has not yet successfully completed an earlier grieving process (Stoddart & McDonnell, 1999).

MOURNING CUSTOMS AND RITUAL

Grief responses involve accepting the loss, experiencing grief, adjusting to an environment without the deceased, withdrawing emotional energy from the relationship, and reinvesting it in new relationships. Some indicators of an individual going through this process may include: behavioral changes, mood changes, isolation, difficulties in relationships, decreased activity, fluctuations in eating and sleeping patterns and difficulties concentrating. These indices are experienced in people with and without developmental disabilities (Stoddart & McDonnell, 1999).

It is well acknowledged by psychologists and professionals in the field of death research, that mourning customs and rituals, particularly participation in the funeral, are powerful and significant means of assisting the bereft person to overcome and handle his grief. Over the ages, different cultures and religions have developed rites and customs that help the mourner express his feelings and get through this critical period as peacefully as possible, while rearranging his life according to the altered reality (Raphael, 1994).

Luchterhand and Murphy (1998) in their book "Helping Adults with Mental Retardation Grieve a Death Loss," stress the special importance of the mourning rituals to the bereaving individual with intellectual disabilities. Why is that so?

It must be emphasized that the cognitive processes of persons with intellectual and other developmental disabilities are generally concrete and they often require tangible and practical expression of a concept or a notion in order to understand its meaning. Given that opportunity and, perhaps, some additional time, we believe that the person with disabilities will be able to sufficiently comprehend most of his life experiences, including the death of a loved one. It is, therefore, of paramount importance that the bereft person with intellectual disabilities be allowed to participate fully in the mourning rituals and practices that are the custom of his family or the culture in which he lives (Koepel & Hollins, 1989).

These rituals may be divided into three categories:

- Rituals performed *with the departed*, such as sitting with body, saying prayers, attending the wake.
- Rituals performed *to mark the passing*, such as obituary columns.
- Prescribed *Social Behavior*, such as wearing black or not wearing make-up.

JEWISH MOURNING RITUALS

Jewish law and tradition are not different from other religions in this regard. Many diverse and detailed customs govern the behavior of the Jewish mourner and those in contact with him or her at this difficult time. An examination of Jewish mourning rituals shows that many of these practices are indeed suitable for the inclusion of individuals with intellectual disabilities and will serve the purpose of assisting them in confronting their loss and grief and grasping the reality of death (Wagschal, 1999). This will be illustrated with a number of examples from our experiences with the study population:

The Funeral

The Jewish traditional funeral is generally attended by many friends and relatives who accompany the deceased on his final journey. Indeed, the Hebrew word for funeral is *Levayah*–which literally means to escort or to accompany. The law (Halacha) requires that the deceased be eulogized and then carried to the grave by participants of the funeral, where he is placed for eternal rest. The person with intellectual disabilities should be encouraged to participate in the funeral and take his place with the other bereaved family members. A brief explanation should help him to understand that he is an active participant in bringing his loved one to his or her resting place and that the deceased feels no pain or suffering. Active participation will increase the probability that the person with intellectual disabilities will paint a realistic picture of the burial process, minimizing misconceptions and anxieties. Two additional rituals, part of the funeral service, emphasize to the individual with disabilities his "mourner status."

First, the *kriyah*–the ritual tearing of the garments–an expression of pain, is done at a point of extreme grief and distress. This is an especially tangible expression of mourning.

Second, the *Shurah*,–after the burial the participants form two parallel lines and as the mourners pass between them, and they are comforted. In this manner, the person with intellectual disabilities is shown to be part of the family–his grief is recognized and legitimate and he too is comforted.

HaShiva–The Seven Days of Mourning

Perhaps the best known Jewish mourning custom, sitting Shiva, involves numerous and detailed manifestations of the mourner's bereavement and hardship. The customs are practical and designed to emphasize and encourage expressions of grief and sorrow. Examples are:

- Sitting on a low seat
- Restrictions of washing oneself
- Refraining from having one's hair cut or shaving
- Refraining from changing into clean clothes or wearing leather shoes
- Refraining from joyous activity

The person with intellectual disabilities will benefit greatly from his participation in the shiva for as long as it is possible. The different manifestations of mourning will allow the person the opportunity to express his personal grief in a fitting manner, while in a sympathetic and supportive environment. Indeed, the Jewish sages have said that crying is the natural way of expressing grief and that the first three days of mourning are the appropriate time for crying.

A further aspect of sitting shiva is the comforting of the mourners by visitors. Sitting shiva creates a unique opportunity for friends (who may also have intellectual disabilities) and professionals to visit and console the bereft individual. Professionals may, for example, remark: "I fully understand how you feel" or "I know how hard it is for you," thereby, helping the person with disabilities understand what is happening to him, and know that it is all right to feel that way.

The Final Example Is the Obituary

In many countries it is customary to publicize a person's passing by placing an obituary in the newspaper. In Israel this is done uniquely by putting up the obituary in the form of a notice, posted at the entrance to the deceased or the mourners' homes, in the neighborhood, and at places of work. In many of our residential settings when a resident suffers the loss of a loved one, the staff will prepare an obituary notice and put it up. In this way the entire resident and staff community may offer their condolences to the bereft individual.

CONCLUSION

Contact with dying and bereavement, unfortunate as it may be, is a critical part of one's formulation of the concept of death. Individuals with intellectual disabilities who during their lifetime experience loss and separation, will be better equipped to handle additional incidents of death and bereavement. It is therefore of extreme importance that these individuals are allowed to take part in ritual practices and customs when experiencing the death of a loved one. Jewish mourning rituals, as a result of their practical and structured nature are seemingly beneficial to bereft individuals with intellectual disabilities, assisting them in confronting their loss and grief and grasping the reality of death.

REFERENCES

Harper, D.C. & Wadsworth, J.S. (1993), Grief in Adults with Mental Retardation: Preliminary Findings, *Research in Developmental Disabilities*, 14, 313-330.
Kloeppel, D.A. & Hollins, S. (1989), Double Handicap: Mental Retardation and Death in the Family, *Death Studies*, 13, 31-38.
Ludlow, B.L., (1999), Life After Loss: Legal Ethical and Practical Issues, In S.S. Herr and G. Weber. (eds.) Aging, Rights and Quality of Life. Baltimore: Paul H. Brookes.
Moise, L.E., (1978), In Sickness and in Death, *Mental Retardation*, 16, 397-398.
Raphael, B. (1994), The Anatomy of Bereavement, Northvale NJ: Jason Aronson.

Seltzer, M.M., (1985), Informal Supports for aging mentally retarded persons, *Americal Journal of Mental Deficiency*, 73, 259-265.

Stoddart, K. & McDonnell, J. (1999), Addressing Grief and Loss in Adults with Developmental Disabilities, *Journal on Developmental Disabilities*, 6(2), 51-65.

Wagschal, S., (1999), Halochos of Aveilus–Laws for the Mourner, Feldheim Publishers, Nanuet: New York.

Bridge Ministries for Disability Concerns:
A Community Ministry Model

Mary Galvin, MTS

SUMMARY. Persons with physical and/or developmental disabilities often find themselves wondering where to look for the support that they need. Moreover, they often find that their loneliness and isolation are far more painful than their disability itself. They are often seeking someone to "come alongside" them, assist them with procuring the resources they need and look more closely at the meaning of life and God's role in their journey. The paper discusses how Bridge Ministries for Disability Concerns, which serves the Puget Sound area, is one model of ministry devoted to doing this. A description of Bridge will be followed by a discussion of its foundation, core values, areas in which it has pioneered, its approach to specific services, as well as its evaluation as a model. *[Article copies available for a fee from The Haworth Document Delivery Service: 1-800-342-9678. E-mail address: <getinfo@haworthpressinc.com> Website: <http://www.HaworthPress.com> © 2001 by The Haworth Press, Inc. All rights reserved.]*

Mary Galvin is Chaplain/Associate, Bridge Ministries for Disability Concerns.

Address correspondence to: Mary Galvin, Bridge Ministries for Disability Concerns, 520-6th Street South, Kirkland, WA 98033-6717 (E-mail: maryg@bridge min.org).

The author would like to acknowledge the founding Executive Director, Rev. Henk Wapstra, the Board of Directors, and the staff of Bridge Ministries for Disability Concerns without whose devotion and deep commitment this ministry would not have been possible.

[Haworth co-indexing entry note]: "Bridge Ministries for Disability Concerns: A Community Ministry Model." Galvin, Mary. Co-published simultaneously in *Journal of Religion, Disability & Health* (The Haworth Pastoral Press, an imprint of The Haworth Press, Inc.) Vol. 5, No. 2/3, 2001, pp. 157-172; and: *Spirituality and Intellectual Disability: International Perspectives on the Effect of Culture and Religion on Healing Body, Mind, and Soul* (eds: William C. Gaventa, Jr. and David L. Coulter) The Haworth Pastoral Press, an imprint of The Haworth Press, Inc., 2001, pp. 157-172. Single or multiple copies of this article are available for a fee from The Haworth Document Delivery Service [1-800-342-9678, 9:00 a.m. - 5:00 p.m. (EST). E-mail address: getinfo@haworthpressinc.com].

157

KEYWORDS. Disability, inclusion, religion, community, resources, church

Elizabeth Barrett Browning once wrote:

> *Earth's crammed with heaven,*
> *And every common bush afire with God;*
> *But only he who sees, takes off his shoes . . .*

(Bolton & Holloway, 1995, p. 232)

It is impossible to be part of the ministry of Bridge and be oblivious to constant encounters with "common bush[es] afire with God." The individuals that Bridge is privileged to serve are conduits of God's presence, bearers of the Good News, witnesses to the many ways in which God can bring new life out of suffering. This is holy ground.

SACRED ENCOUNTERS

- There is the Bridge volunteer who is blind and takes public transportation to read Braille Scripture to a person with cognitive disabilities. He is delighted to have the opportunity to share his gifts with others.
- There is a 40 year old woman with a moderate cognitive disability whose Circle of Friends has supported her in taking her first shaky steps toward her goal of independence. It has been a constant support through her two moves, teaching her how to live on her own and, more importantly, to believe in herself. Her successful transition has given her the courage to get a second job (a few hours on the weekend) to earn more money so she can travel to visit relatives.
- There is the man for whom Bridge is now guardian who was initially non-verbal, depressed, overweight and not relating well with people. Now, after much attention to his whole living situation, Bridge and his caregivers work as a team to see that his needs are addressed so that he no longer finds it necessary to steal or overeat. He also is connected with a counselor and a communication specialist. His whole personality has come alive. Now he smiles, has lost weight, can spell even complicated words on his new communication device. He is surprising everyone with his sophisticated observations, heretofore never shared.

- There is the man with multiple sclerosis whose power scooter had been stolen, preventing him from attending his college classes. A local television community helper contacted Bridge on his behalf. At the time Bridge did not have such a scooter. Three days later one was donated. Not only was this one almost new, it had much more power than the one that had been stolen and it had the needed left hand drive! When the man was presented with the scooter, he wept.
- There is the person with a variety of disabilities who was living alone in a rent-free home with no hot water, very little heat and only a small stipend from a friend. The food provided by a local food bank was sometimes spoiled. The previous year she had tried to apply for government assistance, but had not understood the process, so had not received any help. By the time a Bridge chaplain was contacted and made a home visit, she was deteriorating rapidly both physically and emotionally. Through attentive listening to her story and her discouragement, it became apparent that her faith was a strong support for her. Consequently, it was natural to pray and discuss her faith journey with her as connections with community and church resources were being made. Accompanied this time by someone to assist her, she began to receive some government assistance the day she applied. Other sources of help took more time. Eventually, a caseworker, who was willing to look at her total living situation, was found. At this point Bridge's assistance began to decrease, as resources from others increased. She has since been able to access the medical attention she needs, is living in a good situation, and is looking forward to job training.

These brief *vignettes* represent the heart of Bridge. The Ministry's grounding in Gospel values represents its soul. There are hundreds of stories like the above; open invitations to experience "common bushes afire with God." This is holy ground. These stories illustrate the underlying theology and philosophy of Bridge, which is built on relationships and connections of persons with physical and/or developmental disabilities with the resources they need.

In the following discussion, the reader is invited to look at Bridge as one model of ministry. A description of Bridge will be followed by a discussion of its foundation, core values, areas in which it has pioneered, its approach to specific services, as well as its evaluation as a model.

What Is Bridge Ministries for Disability Concerns?

Bridge is a relational ministry in which listening skills, pastoral care, social services, churches, and advocacy converge. Its Mission Statement reads:

> Bridge Ministries celebrates and honors the God-given dignity and potential of persons with physical and developmental disabilities and their families who are "falling through the cracks" of church and community networks. Bridge serves without discrimination by . . . helping people help themselves; offering hope, encouragement and concrete help; bridging to/networking with church and community.

Bridge serves in a variety of ways specific to the needs of indiviuals with disabilities, their families, and caregivers. In addition, the Ministry partners with churches, the community at large, and its agencies to support and enhance their relationships with persons with disabilities. Bridge accomplishes this by building connections within the community and working with them to increase awareness about needs, but also about the capacities and gifts through which persons with disabilities can enhance all of society, if given the opportunity.

Bridge Ministries is a 501(c)(3) non-profit ministry supported by gifts from individuals, churches, businesses, corporations, and fundraisers. While the Bridge office is located in Kirkland, Washington (near Seattle) the Ministry extends throughout the Puget Sound area. Last year there were 8,000 contacts with or on behalf of the persons Bridge serves.

> The ultimate vision for Bridge will have been realized when persons with disabilities are fully welcomed and included into all communities as valued and contributing members, who themselves are nurtured and who nurture others: physically; spiritually; materially; socially; and emotionally. (A statement from Core Values of Bridge Ministries.)

The Building of Bridge

"Get me outta here. I can't take it anymore!" a voice called out after him as Rev. Hendrik "Henk" Wapstra, a Presbyterian minister, was leaving a nursing home one day after visiting a man in his late 20s. The man's 18-wheeler truck had spun out on black ice, leaving him with quadriplegia. When the man had first arrived at the nursing home he was greeted with, "What are you doing here? We're not equipped to handle quads!" Henk listened carefully to this man and felt he was being called by God to "do something" about this situation. Other "rallying calls that helped to solidify Bridge," according to Henk, were his many friends and parishioners who were also living with disabilities.

By listening to their stories Henk discovered the extent to which persons with disabilities were not getting their needs met: needs that were continuing to increase because of advances in medicine, thus enabling newborns with medical conditions, persons with disabilities and accident survivors to live longer. Gaps in services also existed as students with disabilities transitioned from their high school programs into more independent living situations. Resources were often difficult to find and access. Many persons were finding that it was the isolation, not the disability itself that was causing the greater pain, since connections with natural communities and mainstream society were often non-existent. Meanwhile, inflation, coupled with funding cuts in entitlements, was seriously impacting the services available. Henk also noticed that despite their need for connections, many persons with disabilities were not present in church and community groups (despite the 1994 estimate that persons with disabilities constitute almost 20.6% of the general population) (McNeil, 1997).

It was during a trip to California in 1987 that Henk found himself "wrestling" with God about whether he was being called to found a ministry for persons with disabilities. He made his decision and he began his journey back up the coast toward home. By Los Angeles, Henk had named the ministry; by San Francisco, he had received encouragement and prayer at a Congregational Awareness seminar; by Seattle, he had chosen his start-up Board of Directors. It was in June of 1987 that Henk's visionary leadership, entrepreneurial aptitude, pastoral sensitivity and love for people converged in a ministry that was to take its direction from "needs encountered." Henk remembers that "One step just led to another. It carved its own way."

Through the years the staff has grown to nine. Currently there are: two Chaplains, two Guardianship Associates, a Volunteer Ministries Coordinator, two staff in the Equipment Department, and two staff in Office Administration. The staff itself represents a variety of Christian denominations.

In January of 2000, after thirteen years of guiding Bridge to be the respected ministry it is today and after touching countless lives, Rev. Henk Wapstra decided to retire. His legacy has impacted not only the

Seattle area, but, also, other parts of the country where friends of Bridge would like to have it cloned. Currently Bridge is involved in a search for a new Executive Director.

The Core Values of Bridge

> To love is not to give of your riches but to reveal to others their riches, their gifts, their value and to trust them and their capacity to grow. So it is important to approach people . . . gently, so gently, not forcing yourself upon them, but accepting them as they are, with humility and respect. (Vanier, 1998, p. 80)

In order to support its mission, Bridge is committed to the following core values.

- It is a relational ministry that arises from a Christian commitment that is rooted in Christ's ministry with persons who were marginalized.
- It strives to promote hope in the context of Jesus' words, "I came that they might have life and have it abundantly" (John 10:10 *RSV*).
- It advocates for the full participation of persons with disabilities in the life of church and society for the mutual enrichment and benefit of all.
- It "comes alongside" persons and respects their life journeys, regardless of their religious beliefs or cultural differences.
- It responds in freedom, love and acceptance, knowing that it is called to be responsible *to* the persons it serves, not *for* them.
- It recognizes that it is not Bridge's responsibility to "fix" individuals, but to honor and value them in ways that encourage them to use their gifts and to discern for themselves God's action in their lives.
- It respects confidentiality.
- It celebrates the mutuality of relationships among all people.
- It shows respect for individuals seeking the assistance of Bridge by referring to them as "persons we serve," rather than the more impersonal designation of "client." Care is also taken to avoid the pejorative connotation of "the disabled" or "the handicapped." The focus is the human being who happens to have a disability.
- It acknowledges the wisdom and the often prophetic way in which persons with disabilities can grace the lives of others, reminding

them that, in fact, their very "imperfection is . . . the crack in the armor, the 'wound' that lets God in." (Kurtz & Ketcham, 1992, p. 28)

By listening attentively to persons with physical and/or developmental disabilities, others often find themselves challenged to rethink the priorities that society holds dear; priorities such as physical beauty, intelligence, material possessions, independence, and freedom. Temporarily able-bodied persons come to admire the grace with which many persons with disabilities choose to deal with their circumstances. The importance of authentic relationship in the lives of the individuals Bridge serves calls forth the building of community for which society hungers.

Furthermore, individuals living with disabilities often remind others about God's call to slow down in this fast-paced world, so that they can be present to the moment and truly be with the individual whose pace is far more attuned to the injunction, "Be still, and know that I am God." (Ps. 46:10 *RSV*) In this way persons with disabilities are called to spend time reflecting on their own thirst for spirituality.

What Makes Bridge a Pioneering Model of Ministry?

Bridge is a pioneering model of ministry in three key ways: it is a community-based ministry; it uses an integrated approach to serving; it is available to act in the interim, in the breach, before connections to other resources can be made.

Community-Based: At the time that Bridge was conceived in 1987, "community-based chaplaincy" represented an evolving understanding and approach to ministry. The term "community-based" means that the broader community is the locus of service, not a particular congregation, or a hospital, or an institution per se. This changing landscape of ministry offers the opportunity to stay connected with an individual in his/her environment as needed, until a natural conclusion is reached.

Integrated Approach: Bridge has an integrated approach to serving individuals, church and community. It is neither totally church-based, nor totally secular. Rather it walks comfortably in many arenas, while acknowledging its foundation in Gospel values. It interfaces with social service, government, medical and business communities, as well as with churches. Therefore, Bridge has a broad base from which to minister and is not limited to providing only one or two services.

Two corollaries flow from this fact:

- Bridge is in a position to effect change in both church and community. Its funding sources allow it the freedom to respond to a variety of needs. Referrals come from caseworkers, pastors, nurses, physical and occupational therapists, counselors, other disability organizations, and word of mouth.
- Because it is an ecumenical Christian organization, Bridge can access many different denominations in order to advocate on behalf of persons with disabilities.

Available in the Interim: The Ministry is a safety net, when there's no one else to bridge the gap in services and support; before a person with a physical and/or developmental disability is connected with his/her case worker, pastor, housing, friend to visit, or other resources. Bridge is there to accompany a person on his/her journey as long as there remains a need for advocacy, pastoral care, or other support.

This relationship with Bridge may ebb and flow throughout the course of a person's lifetime as he/she encounters changes in life, many of which are losses. Sometimes transitions are very difficult and seem insurmountable. It is important for the person to know that he/she is not alone and that Bridge will be there if it is needed. The freedom to talk about God, if the person indicates an interest, while also working in a secular environment on concrete resources enables ministry to happen on a variety of levels. The key is to recognize and facilitate the balance between support and independence.

The Translation of Values into Services

The following are the key areas of ministry in which Bridge is engaged. Each one exemplifies the mission, core values, philosophy and theology discussed above. While many of the types of services that Bridge provides are available through various organizations, the following discussion will highlight the ways in which they have been integrated at Bridge.

Not surprisingly, given Bridge's emphasis on the importance of relationship, each of its ministries is person focused, not program focused per se. Although, in describing its work, Bridge might refer to its "programs," it is really the staff members who are "the program." The emphasis is always on the individual/organization seeking assistance and how the services of Bridge can be tailored to accommodate particular needs. Whatever the entry point might be, the staff tries to be aware of additional ways in which Bridge might serve a given person or organization.

Basic Services

Bridge provides four basic categories of service, including Chaplaincy, Legal Guardianship, Durable Medical Equipment and the Volunteer Ministries Program.

CHAPLAINCY

Pastoral care is an important aspect of the ministry of Bridge. As chaplains encounter the persons Bridge serves, they pray that God will bless their presence, actions and words so that, hopefully, they will become conduits of God's affirming love and hope to the persons they are serving.

By taking the time to visit individuals with physical and/or developmental disabilities in their homes and eliminating transportation worries, Bridge conveys to the persons seeking assistance that it takes their concerns seriously. It is a way of showing respect for individuals who very often feel ostracized from society and who see themselves as having very little worth. Requests for service might include: information and referral; accompaniment for a time on a person's spiritual journey; support through difficult losses; involvement of more people in their lives; or simply offering respect and appreciation for them as human beings and a sense of hope for the future.

While Bridge chaplains are not social workers, they are available to persons with physical and/or developmental disabilities in the interim until connections can be made with social workers or whatever resources may be needed. For example, chaplains not only suggest possible resources to persons, but they often help them through the complex maze of connecting with those resources. During this process, the chaplain can minister with the person in additional ways that respect the personal spiritual struggles that can arise during life changes. Chaplains often assist in locating the documentation required; accompanying persons to interviews to support and advocate on their behalf; and assuring that they are able to keep the doctor appointments that are required to qualify for help. Frequently someone needs to assume the role of advocate and smooth the way until the individual begins receiving the benefits to which he/she is entitled.

Church partnerships, another important part of the ministry of Bridge chaplains, will be discussed in the section entitled "On-Going Links to Church and Community."

LEGAL GUARDIANSHIPS

There are a number of guardianship services available in the community. The following is a description of the approach used by Bridge. This program was developed in response to requests for guardianship on behalf of persons with developmental disabilities who have little or no family involvement, few assets, and who would otherwise be "wards of the state."

As is true of the ministry of Bridge in general, the focus of this program is to help the persons for whom Bridge is guardian to live life to the fullest extent possible. Therefore, the two guardianship administrators (who are on call 24 hours a day, seven days a week) visit each of the 44 persons in Bridge's guardianship "family," at least monthly to build relationships and to go on outings to their favorite places. This allows the guardianship administrator to oversee an individual's well-being, living arrangement, church affiliation (if they choose to have one), employment, the standard of care being provided, any change in the person's behavior and medical situation, and to work collaboratively with the team of care providers. Often visits are more frequent than once a month, such as when a person is hospitalized, when there is a birthday, or when a relative whom Bridge has reconnected with a person comes to town for a visit, etc. To the extent possible, every major event in the person's life is celebrated.

It is a privilege to see human beings begin to blossom when they are moved into the least restrictive (yet appropriately supervised) living environment. This allows them to have greater interaction with their community where they are afforded more choices, an opportunity to learn who they are as individuals, and elevated self esteem. Stories of new life abound in these settings.

DURABLE MEDICAL EQUIPMENT

Since its inception, Bridge has given away $1,500,000 worth of donated durable medical equipment. Last year alone the total was $280,000. (This is based on the original cost.) This program has become even more important since some local agencies have opted not to handle such equipment anymore, thus reducing the number of resources available. Bridge takes in donations of used durable medical equipment (e.g., wheelchairs, scooters, walkers, commodes, and shower chairs), cleans and restores it with the help of its team of dedicated volunteers, and then distributes it free of charge to persons who could not otherwise afford it.

Procuring such equipment that is often not covered by other funding resources can have an astounding impact on a person's life. Whether it is in-home equipment that makes life easier or varying modes of transportation, durable medical equipment can open up whole new vistas of hope and community access to someone who had previously been a virtual prisoner in his/her own home. The need for this ministry is so great that equipment waiting lists to procure equipment are often long. This is one of the most heavily used services that Bridge provides. Requests in this area often involve links with other services as well.

VOLUNTEER MINISTRIES

The Mission Statement of the Volunteer Ministries Program reads: "In supporting the mission of Bridge, we are committed to building relationships between persons with disabilities and volunteers that unleash and celebrate their God-given gifts" (Bridge Ministries, 2000). This program establishes two-way bridges that nurture and celebrate both persons with disabilities *and* volunteers, thus facilitating an important community connection for both. Particularly for the person with a disability, who may be experiencing a real relationship with someone from the community for the first time, this opportunity can represent a fullness of life heretofore unattained.

Volunteer participation (which includes both individuals with physical and/or developmental disabilities, as well as others in the community) also enriches and expands Bridge's capacity to address the diverse needs of the Ministry. Bridge's 206 volunteers are involved in friend-to-friend visiting, Circles of Friends, on-call response opportunities, group events, and office support.

Other On-Going Links to Church and Community

Bridge provides seven services that are on-going links to the community, including community based Circles of Friends, church partnerships, church-based Circles of Friends, Bridge to Love phone ministry, education, the *Connections Newsletter,* and Bridge's website.

COMMUNITY BASED CIRCLES OF FRIENDS

A Circle of Friends is a gathering of individuals around a person with a disability (focus person) in order to support his/her goals and dreams. This is another example of a bridge designed for two-way traffic. Circles are sacred because they honor and respect the God-given dignity of the person for whom the Circle is called, helping to alleviate feelings of low self esteem and worthlessness, by focusing on capacity. In the majority of cases Circles make a significant difference in the lives of all involved, but especially for the focus persons. Each Circle is unique because everyone's goals and dreams are different. Some Circles are purely social. Others deal with a variety of topics such as housing, independent living skills, employment, or family issues. Circle members are not asked to solve all the problems in an individual's life. Oftentimes it is simply their help with brainstorming and just "being there" that enables new possibilities to surface and engenders hope. Members of Circles often find it comforting to know that other people are also involved in assisting the person who has a disability and that their participation is based on what is possible for them.

Circles promote safety in two ways. (1) They are forums in which focus persons can be free to express who they are, without fear of judgment. (2) They can also be a means of protection for a person living alone with only a couple of caregivers. Just knowing that a group of people is involved in the life of an individual who has a disability can be an effective deterrent to potential abuse by a caregiver, as well as a vehicle for advocacy.

Circles are made possible through the efforts of facilitators and Circle members working in conjunction with the focus person. Bridge recruits, trains, mentors and provides monthly meeting support for facilitators.

Although the notion of "circles" has probably existed since the cave dwellers sat around the campfire at night and shared their lives with each other, this present day version is dramatically changing the lives of persons with disabilities, as well as the Circle members. Community calls forth life for everyone.

CHURCH PARTNERSHIPS

Many persons who have disabilities are missing from our congregations. Because Bridge is ecumenical, it is free to minister with churches representing many different denominations, exploring how to most effectively partner with them to welcome persons with disabilities into their congregations, realizing that to the extent that persons with disabilities are absent from our churches, the Body of Christ is incomplete. Individuals sometimes request that a Bridge staff member accompany them on an initial visit to the pastor or outreach minister of a church and to participate in the exploration of how they might mutually enrich one another. Such consultation often results in imaginative ways in which existing church structures can incorporate persons with disabilities and share in each others' gifts. Collaboration with churches ahead of time enables them to have a basis for response within their own communities.

Bridge staff is frequently invited to speak at churches, regarding the services it provides. It also does awareness presentations in which simulation exercises are followed by discussion of what it means to have a disability or how to interact with someone who does.

An outgrowth of the informal mentoring Bridge now does with a variety of churches is a proposed partnership whereby Bridge chaplains work with churches for one year to help them become more pro-active and self-sufficient in their ministry with persons with disabilities.

OTHER LINKING SERVICES

These include: Church-Based Circles of Friends (through which faith communities can become more involved); Bridge to Love Phone Ministry (whereby persons with disabilities offer phone support to others); education (through awareness seminars, conferences and workshops). Oftentimes the individuals served are invited by the Bridge presenters to accompany them in these educational efforts, since they are the real experts who are living with disabilities. Bridge's quarterly *Connections Newsletter* and its website *bridgemin.org* also promote on-going links.

Special Events

Bridge also provides special events to provide networking opportunities among the persons it serves, church and community. Monthly

Sunday Evening Celebrations are one key way in which Bridge involves several area churches in concrete opportunities to co-host dinners for persons with disabilities from their own congregations and neighborhoods, as well as for the persons Bridge serves.

The annual "Walk 'n Roll a-thon" is designed to be both a fundraiser and a way to celebrate the persons Bridge serves. Ferryboat rides provide fun and live entertainment on Puget Sound for the persons for whom Bridge is guardian, while the annual Overnight Camp is a highly anticipated and well-attended yearly event to celebrate community.

EVALUATION OF BRIDGE AS A MODEL OF MINISTRY

What Gives This Model Life?

- The Ministry is rooted in a strong Christian commitment and a fidelity to the core values listed above.
- It offers community-based chaplaincy that is not tied to an institution.
- Bridge uses an integrated approach to serving a person's physical, spiritual, material, social and emotional needs, as well as serving church and community in relation to persons with disabilities. Therefore, Bridge has the freedom to respond to "needs encountered" in many areas, not just one or two.
- It is there in the interim when there's no one else to bridge the gap in services and support.
- Because it is interdenominational, Bridge is in a unique position to have entree to a variety of churches, thereby multiplying its effectiveness in partnering, educating and advocating on behalf of persons with physical and/or developmental disabilities.
- It is a touchstone throughout the life of a person with a disability as his/her needs ebb and flow.
- Its non-restrictive funding sources free the Ministry to be where it is needed.
- Collaboration and creative problem-solving are encouraged in all aspects of ministry, thus encouraging openness to new possibilities.
- There is a deep commitment to the mission of Bridge by each Board and staff member because the work of Bridge is a ministry, a vocation. The same sense of collaboration that Bridge values in its relationships with the persons it serves is at work among the staff.

What Is Challenging About This Model?

- Funding is an ongoing challenge for Bridge as it is for many nonprofits. Bridge has envisioned many additional avenues of service that can only be implemented by adding several more staff and a larger facility.
- It would be helpful to have a social worker on staff who could help with connections to government and social service resources. This would allow the chaplains more time to focus on more traditional aspects of pastoral care, to build more connections with church and community members, and permit them to devote more time to nurturing the potential and gifts of persons with disabilities.
- Another challenge posed by this model of ministry is the discernment of the role of Bridge in a given situation and the degree of involvement that is appropriate. How can Bridge best partner with the individuals and organizations it serves, providing support without fostering dependence?
- As in any area of human services, there is always a danger of burnout. There are so many needs and never enough time to adequately meet them all. A caregiver in whatever capacity can begin to feel overwhelmed and lose a sense of perspective and passion for his/her calling. Prayerful reflection and careful discernment, along with a clear sense of the boundaries of this Ministry, are needed to prevent overwork and burnout.
- As in any business or ministry, there is the on-going need to revisit the theological roots, the core values and the growth of Bridge in order to evaluate its continuing effectiveness in light of the needs of individuals with disabilities, church and community.

CONCLUSION

The focus of this paper has been to describe Bridge Ministries for Disability Concerns as one model of ministry that serves persons with physical and/or developmental disabilities. Although other organizations for persons with disabilities provide services similar to those of Bridge, the approach to the paper has been to identify the ways in which Bridge interprets and integrates its approach to ministry. It provides community-based pastoral care with a focus on integration of services and is designed to respond in "the interim" before connections to resources have been made. It has the freedom to interface with both church and secular communities, while maintaining its commitment to Gospel values.

The foregoing has been only one lens through which to view this Ministry. There are many others, the most important of which are the stories of the persons whom Bridge is privileged to serve. They are the occasion of daily encounters with "common bush[es]afire with God." They are the reason for all the visioning and excitement as Bridge looks forward to a future in which persons with physical and/or developmental disabilities will be *"fully welcomed and included into all communities as valued and contributing members, who themselves are nurtured and who nurture others: physically; spiritually; materially; socially; and emotionally"* (a statement from "Core Values of Bridge Ministries").

AUTHOR NOTE

Since 1993, Mary Galvin has been a Chaplain/Associate with Bridge Ministries for Disability Concerns. She holds a Master of Theological Studies degree from Seattle University and Master of Library Science degree from the University of Washington. Mary is certified by the National Association of Catholic Chaplains. She has conducted a study entitled "In Quest of the 'Seamless Garment': A Study of Ministry with Persons with Disabilities in the Archdiocese of Seattle." Before coming to Bridge, Mary was chaplain at Fircrest School, a residential facility for persons with developmental disabilities. Prior to that, she worked as a librarian for Seattle Public Library. She is married and has two children.

REFERENCES

Browning, E. B. (1995). *Aurora Leigh and Other Poems*. New York, NY: Penguin Books.
Harper Study Bible Revised Standard Version. (1971). Grand Rapids, MI: Zondervan.
Kurtz, E. & Ketcham, K. (1992). *The Spirituality of Imperfection*. New York, NY: Bantam.
U.S. Bureau of the Census. (1997). *Current Population Reports* (1994-1995). Washington, DC: U.S. Government Printing Office.
Vanier, J. (1988). *The Broken Body*. New York, NY: Paulist Press.

Index

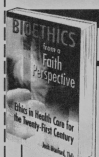

TO ORDER: CALL: 1-800-429-6784 / FAX: 1-800-895-0582 (Outside US/Canada: + 607-771-0012) / E-MAIL: orders@haworthpressinc.com

☐ YES, please send me **Bioethics From a Faith Perspective**

____ in soft at $19.95 ISBN: 0-7890-1510-2.
____ in hard at $49.95 ISBN: 0-7890-1509-9.

- Individual orders outside US, Canada, and Mexico must be prepaid by check or credit card.
- Discounts are not available on 5+ text prices and not available in conjunction with any other discount. • Discount not applicable on books priced under $15.00.
- 5+ text prices are not available for jobbers and wholesalers.
- Postage & handling: in US: $4.00 for first book; $1.50 for each additional book.
  Outside US: $5.00 for first book; $2.00 for each additional book.
- Canadian residents: please add appropriate sales tax after postage & handling. Canadian residents: please add 7% GST after postage & handling. Canadian residents of Newfoundland, Nova Scotia, and New Brunswick, also add 8% for province tax. • Payment in UNESCO coupons welcome.
- If paying in Canadian dollars, use current exchange rate to convert to US dollars.
- Please allow 3-4 weeks for delivery after publication.
- Prices and discounts subject to change without notice.

Signature _____

☐ **BILL ME LATER** ($5 service charge will be added).
(Not available for individuals outside US/Canada/Mexico. Service charge is waived for/jobbers/wholesalers/booksellers.)

☐ Check here if billing address is different from shipping address and attach purchase order and billing address information.

☐ **PAYMENT ENCLOSED $** _____
(Payment must be in US or Canadian dollars by check or money order drawn on a US or Canadian bank.)

☐ **PLEASE BILL MY CREDIT CARD:**

☐ AmEx ☐ Diners Club ☐ Discover ☐ Eurocard ☐ JCB ☐ Master Card ☐ Visa

Account Number _____

Expiration Date _____

Signature _____

THE HAWORTH PRESS, INC., 10 Alice Street, Binghamton, NY 13904-1580 USA

Please complete the information below or tape your business card in this area.

NAME _____

INSTITUTION _____

ADDRESS _____

CITY _____

STATE _____ ZIP _____

COUNTRY _____

COUNTY (NY residents only) _____

E-MAIL _____

May we use your e-mail address for confirmations and other types of information? ( ) Yes ( ) No We appreciate receiving your e-mail address and fax number. Haworth would like to e-mail or fax special discount offers to you, as a preferred customer. We will never share, rent, or exchange your e-mail address or fax number. We regard such actions as an invasion of your privacy.

☐ YES, please send me **Bioethics From a Faith Perspective (ISBN: 0-7890-1510-2)** to consider on a 60-day no risk examination basis. I understand that I will receive an invoice payable within 60 days, or that if I decide to adopt the book, my invoice will be cancelled. I understand that I will be billed at the lowest price. (60-day offer available only to teaching faculty in US, Canada, and Mexico / Outside US/ Canada, a proforma invoice will be sent upon receipt of your request and must be paid in advance of shipping. A full refund will be issued with proof of adoption.)

This information is needed to process your examination copy order.

Signature _____

Course Title(s) _____

Current Text(s) _____

Enrollment _____

Semester _____ Decision Date _____

Office Tel _____ Hours _____

(09) (15)   02/02   BIC03

FAX